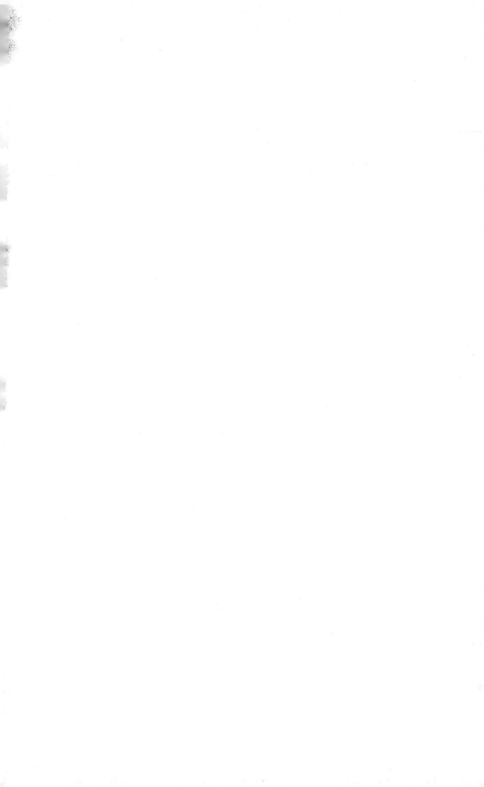

EVERYTHING YOU WANT TO KNOW ABOUT COSMETICS

Other books by Toni Stabile

Cosmetics: The Great American Skin Game
Cosmetics: Trick or Treat?

cos·met′ic [Gr. *kosmetikos* skilled in decorating, fr. *kosmos* order, ornament.]—n. Any preparation (except soap) to be applied to the surface of the human body for lending attractiveness, for theatrical make-up, or for cleansing or conditioning the skin, hair, nails, etc.

—*Webster*

cosmetic (1) articles intended to be rubbed, poured, sprinkled, or sprayed on, introduced into, or otherwise applied to the human body or any part thereof for cleansing, beautifying, promoting attractiveness, or altering the appearance, and (2) articles intended for use as a component of any such articles: except that such term shall not include soap.

—*Food, Drug, and Cosmetic Act*

EVERYTHING YOU WANT TO KNOW ABOUT COSMETICS*

*Or What Your Friendly Clerk Didn't Tell You

Toni Stabile

DODD, MEAD & COMPANY   New York

Special acknowledgment is made to Ann Landers, the New York *Daily News,* and Field Newspaper Syndicate for permission to use the copyrighted Ann Landers column.

Copyright © 1984 by Toni Stabile
All rights reserved
No part of this book may be reproduced in any form
without permission in writing from the publisher.
Published by Dodd, Mead & Company, Inc.
79 Madison Avenue, New York, N.Y. 10016
Distributed in Canada by
McClelland and Stewart Limited, Toronto
Manufactured in the United States of America
Designed by Levavi & Levavi
First Edition

Library of Congress Cataloging in Publication Data:

Stabile, Toni.
    Everything you want to know about cosmetics, or, What your friendly clerk didn't tell you.

    Bibliography:
    Includes index.
    1. Cosmetics. I. Title.
TP983.S83   1984   363.1'96   84-1514
ISBN 0-396-08358-7

To my parents and family who not only helped along the way but provided me with my most dependable safety net.

Contents

Acknowledgments

Since this book is a distillation of twenty-five years of questioning and probing, it is impossible to acknowledge and thank all those who have made my report possible.

I am indebted to many who prefer to remain anonymous, to countless numbers of consumers, and to those in the various segments of government and industry, all of whom contributed in their special way.

I am especially indebted to Donald A. Davis, editor of *Drug & Cosmetic Industry,* John A. Wenninger, deputy director of the Division of Cosmetics Technology of the Food and Drug Administration, E. Edward Kavanaugh, president of The Cosmetic, Toiletry and Fragrance Association, and Dr. Dennis M. Stark, director of the Laboratory Animal Research Center at The Rockefeller University, for their most generous cooperation, their time, interest, and their valued help. To my editor, Evan Marshall, my appreciation for his encouragement and his light, sure touch in editing my manuscript. And to my brother, Vincent, for his all-around help and forbearance.

EVERYTHING YOU WANT TO KNOW ABOUT COSMETICS

— 1 —
So You Don't Use Cosmetics?

At any given time, the average customer is using
between 11 and 12 cosmetics.
—**Survey,**
Food and Drug Administration

You're one of those lucky ones, you say. Your ancestors willed you good looks and a nearly flawless skin, so you don't use cosmetics. Neither does your husband or your children, if they're part of your household—or your father and mother, sister, brother, grandfather, grandmother, boyfriend, girl friend . . . Take your pick, and chances are you'll be wrong. Just about everyone in the civilized world is a cosmetic user. As for those to whom civilization has yet to thrust its assembly lines, they've no doubt arrived at their own forms of cosmetics, courtesy of their kindly witch doctor or local Helena Rubinstein.

In our world, cosmetics await our very entrance into it. We're baby-oiled and baby-powdered and baby-lotioned and baby-shampooed to a fare-thee-well. Male and female, we continue through life accompanied by tons of toothpaste, sham-

1

poo, bubble bath, talcum powder, deodorants, suntan oils, sunscreen lotions, mouthwash, foot powder, baby oil, hair conditioners, hand lotions, and lip protectors.

But, you say, those aren't cosmetics; those are everyday necessities for family grooming. They're shopping-list items. Maybe they're toiletries or grooming items, but "cosmetics" are makeup—lipstick, rouge, eye shadow . . .

Actually, the powder and paint of cosmetics represents a minuscule part of the multibillion dollars that Americans alone spend on cosmetics. Every product every member of the family uses every day to cleanse, groom, beautify, or otherwise alter the appearance—except soap—is classified as a cosmetic.

If you've succumbed to buying some of the lines of dog shampoos and grooming products, even the family pet has joined us as a cosmetic consumer. Some horses long ago became consumers when Elizabeth Arden rubbed down her horses' legs with her cream.

Even after at least part of us has left this world, we're not likely to escape. Every mortician has a makeup kit at the ready to simulate the blush of life on the lifeless. Some have makeup artists who specialize in the art. Most are on call on a free-lance basis.

Macho men, who wouldn't knowingly be caught dead with makeup and who will vehemently deny using cosmetics, nevertheless contribute to the total amount of fragrance used by the male population, which surpasses the amount used by the female population. Reason: Fragrance is part of shaving creams and after-shave lotions habitually used by many, in addition to shampoo, hair-grooming products, deodorants, talc, suntan lotions, and sunscreens.

The growing list of colognes and esoteric cosmetics designed to beckon more dollars from recalcitrant men is bound to keep the male fragrance consumption ahead of the female's.

QUESTIONS AND ANSWERS

Is it true that Ralph Nader doesn't use cosmetics?

Ralph Nader allowed a television makeup artist to slap some makeup on his face before facing the cameras after he realized how dark his beard looked on the screen. In real life, he says he uses baking soda instead of toothpaste to brush his teeth, and plain soap instead of shaving cream and shampoo to shave his offending beard and wash his good thick hair.

If Ralph Nader uses any products that can be classified as cosmetics, they're minimal, if at all. Mr. Nader may well be the noncosmetic user to prove the rule.

A number of years ago, a big fuss was made because a television personality admitted he didn't use the product he was advertising. Do the people promoting cosmetics actually use the products they promote?

Mostly, the makeup you see on the models, used in advertisements and commercials, is the advertised makeup applied by a professional makeup artist. Whether the model uses that brand of cosmetics away from that particular camera is open to question. I know of no mandate that would force a model to use a particular brand in real life. A popular model could sit for a dozen magazine covers, for instance, and be made up in more than that number of cosmetic lines. Many models are very cost-conscious of the cosmetics they use and buy the least expensive products that they feel will fill their requirements.

As for the so-called "miracle" creams, lotions, and potions heavily promoted for "cell rejuvenation," the "moisturizing miracles" and "scientific breakthroughs" that promise to restore the bloom of youth, it takes little imagination to realize that the barely-out-of-their-teens models used to illustrate the promised results have no need or practical use for the products.

There seem to be mostly men controlling the cosmetic companies and industry. Do you think they're true believers in the products they bring to market? In other words, do they use their own products and do they bring them home to their families to use?

Those are questions only each of the many men who control the cosmetic industry can answer. At least two men in high places admit they don't use antiperspirants or deodorants. One uses baking soda instead because he's allergic to the ingredients in antiperspirants and deodorants. The other claims he doesn't need them because he doesn't sweat.

Whether the manufacturers of the lead-containing hair color "restorers" bring their products home without being positive that no child in the household has access to them is an excellent question to be asked.

What difference does it make if family staples such as toothpaste, shampoo, baby powder, and suntan oils are called cosmetics or over-the-counter preparations, such as the patent medicines we buy?

There's a big difference. Classified as cosmetics, hundreds of thousands of products, routinely used by the entire population, escape most of the consumer safeguards we've come to expect of our foods and drugs.

Doesn't the Federal Food, Drug, and Cosmetic Act cover cosmetics?

The Food, Drug, and Cosmetic Act is an unequal act that exempts cosmetics from most of its regulations.

— 2 —
Is Somebody Down Here Watching?

The problem today is not so much the products
that are known to harm, but the cosmetics that
are not known to be safe.
—**Winton B. Rankin,**
Former Deputy Commissioner,
Food and Drug Administration

Of course, someone or some agency checks cosmetics or toiletries or the everyday grooming products we're using to see that what goes on the store shelves is safe and pure and all that. True?

Unfortunately, not only does the general buying public assume that some of the multiple agencies in Washington look after our well-being with safeguards that prevent harmful or unfit cosmetic products from coming to market, so did the head of a dermatological section of a large hospital.

Hardly known and unpublicized is the fact that, although "Cosmetics" was added in 1938 to the existing food and drug law in the Federal Food, Drug, and Cosmetic (FD&C) Act, the food and drug regulations crumble before they reach the "Cosmetic" appendage.

There is virtually nothing to prevent a harmful cosmetic from reaching the market and millions of consumers. Anyone can put together a bathtub batch of a "new miracle discovery" and hawk it as a cosmetic. Until it is sold in interstate commerce, the Food and Drug Administration cannot act against it even if it is known to be harmful.

According to Heinz J. Eiermann, director of FDA's Division of Cosmetics Technology, the FD&C Act prohibits the marketing of cosmetics that are adulterated or misbranded, as well as their adulteration or misbranding, while in interstate commerce. However, there is no statutory requirement that cosmetic products be proved safe, as is the case with new drugs, or that the truthfulness of cosmetic labeling be substantiated before cosmetics are introduced into interstate commerce. There is also no requirement that cosmetic ingredients, with the exception of color additives, be tested for safety.

Manufacturers or distributors are not required to register their manufacturing establishments, product formulations, or consumer reports of adverse reactions with the FDA, or make available other information on their products.

Mr. Eiermann pointed out that the burden of proof that a cosmetic is adulterated or misbranded rests with the agency. "If we want to remove a cosmetic from the market for lack of safety or for deception, we can do so only by showing that the product is harmful or that its labeling or packaging is false or misleading. If we want to prohibit the further use of an ingredient, we must demonstrate that the ingredient may be poisonous or deleterious under the intended conditions of use."

The general public assumption of cosmetic regulation and consumer safeguards, however, is in sharp contrast to the facts as outlined by the director.

A national survey, conducted in 1980 and 1981, found that 88 percent of the consumers questioned believed that cosmetic manufacturers are required by law to test their products. Ninety-seven percent believed the manufacturers *should* test their products, and about the same number thought that cosmetic firms had to or should submit their data to the government for approval.

Dr. Arthur Hull Hayes, Jr., while he was commissioner of food and drugs, conceded, "These consumer expectations are fulfilled for food and color additives and for drugs—but for cosmetics they are not."

After a cosmetic is sold across state lines and is found to be mislabeled or deleterious, the FDA can attempt to remove the product from the market. If the cosmetic is merely guilty of misleading or deceptive labeling, the FDA can make only one seizure. If the cosmetic is found to be deleterious and is capable of causing harm or has injured, the FDA may make multiple seizures and attempt to get as much of the product off the market as quickly as possible.

Recalls, which are a more efficient way of getting the product out of circulation quickly, usually are at the discretion of the distributing company. It is then still up to the government agency to prove that the cosmetic was mislabeled or injurious.

Legal footwork and foot-dragging can allow the product to remain in the marketplace until the supply is exhausted and the company is ready to introduce a new version of the product. Recent years have seen offending companies also given the option of informing—*or not informing*—consumers of cosmetics considered deleterious by the FDA.

Since the Federal Trade Commission has been practically muzzled and, at times, even threatened with abolition, cosmetic advertising has exploded with claims that would have alerted even the sleepiest of agencies being kept alive with our taxes to protect us from fraudulent and deceptive advertising.

Glossy ads tell us of scientific breakthroughs, medical discoveries, and newly discovered ancient beauty secrets. Television commercials dance by with so many claims for so many miraculous moisturizers that, if the claims are to be believed, a devoted consumer might end up with a face resembling a wet sponge. Emboldened by the anything-goes climate in advertising, some of the exaggerated and unsubstantiated claims are sliding onto cosmetic labels, which are in FDA's territory.

The trend toward "cosmetic quackery" was noted by Commissioner Hayes and explained as "that consumer deception resulting from false or misleading labeling of cosmetics.

"We have seen an increasing number of cosmetics making claims that go far beyond what is generally considered 'cosmetic puffery.' " According to Commissioner Hayes, "We are concerned about claims that are therapeutic in nature.

"The deciding factor in determining the intended use of a product is how most consumers perceive claims made about it. Therefore, if a large number of consumers perceive that a product, on the basis of its label statements and other representations made about it, is intended to prevent or treat disease or otherwise affect the structure or functions of the human body, that product may well be classified as a drug. (This classification may be in addition to its status as a cosmetic.) The question then remaining would become whether it is a prescription or an over-the-counter drug, a new drug or a 'not new' drug, or an adulterated or misbranded drug. If a drug is a new drug, the marketer carries the burden of proving that it is safe and effective before it enters the channels of distribution.

"Although our primary aim in consumer protection has always been product safety, the law also requires us to protect consumers from misbranded products. We have the statutory authority to use discretion in law enforcement, just as the police officer need not give a ticket to every motorist exceeding a given speed limit. If one motorist drives too fast, however, or if too many exceed the speed limit on a certain stretch of the road, ticketing usually is not far behind."

Of the agencies charged with somewhat policing cosmetics, the Post Office can be the fastest, most efficient policeman. Once alerted to fraudulent cosmetic products with deceptive claims and outright frauds, the Post Office can drive the offenders out of the mail and cut off their vital and, often, only link to potential customers. However, the chase usually begins again when the company and products reappear newly named with recycled claims and schemes along with a new post office box number.

With so few consumer safeguards afforded us by those in Washington and environs, consumers, who have come to enjoy and even to appreciate cosmetic and grooming products, are left to wonder why products that outsell over-the-counter patent medicines and prescription drugs combined, and are casually used by the entire population, should be overlooked instead of overseen.

QUESTIONS AND ANSWERS

Why did it take Congress until 1938 to add Cosmetics to the Food, Drug, and Cosmetic Act?

Congress declined to take cosmetics seriously—as much of Congress continues to do—when they were proposed as part of the drug category when the first Pure Food and Drug Law was introduced. Cosmetics were then dropped by the largely male Congress—as it continues to be today—before the law was passed in 1906.

Only after decades of injuries and deaths from cosmetics—and, in particular, a horrendous blinding and death from Lash Lure, a caustic eyebrow and eyelash dye—did Congress awaken to the need to consider any legislation that recognized products that were neither food nor drugs but nevertheless had become part of the household and family shopping list.

What is the situation in Congress now? Is there any new legislation being considered for cosmetics?

There's an apparent stalemate in Congress on cosmetic legislation. Despite testimony that zeroed in on hair dyes and carcinogenic and mutagenic ingredients in cosmetics during the hearings on cancer-causing chemicals called by the House Interstate and Foreign Commerce Subcommittee on Oversight and Investigation in 1978, no bills have seen any action in Congress since the Senate passed and then let die Senator Thomas F. Eagleton's Cosmetic Safety bill in 1980.

What are the prospects for further legislation?

Dim, unless voters become vigilant enough to alert their senators and representatives to the need for legislation to require cosmetic companies to adequately test their products *before* they go to market rather than post-testing the cosmetics on the paying public after they're on the market.

Dr. Arthur Hull Hayes, Jr., who was listed as "Commissioner of Food and Drugs" with no mention of cosmetics since Cosmetics was shoved into the Bureau of Foods and hidden like a poor relative unworthy of its own habitat, admitted, "In spite of the impressive advances in science and technology as well as in consumer awareness, Congress has repeatedly seen no reason to amend the cosmetic provision of the FD&C Act as it has with respect to food and color additives, drugs, and medical devices."

At the same time, Dr. Hayes cited a survey that found that "at any given time the average consumer is using between

11 and 12 cosmetics. Many pounds of products per year are 'rubbed, poured, sprinkled or sprayed on, introduced into, or otherwise applied to the human body,' to quote the FD&C Act. It has been estimated that the number of cosmetic vehicle and fragrance ingredients [used by the cosmetic industry] has grown to about 8,000 chemical entities. [Cosmetic] products consist of at least 25,000 formulations and more than 50,000 brand names. Obviously, the magnitude of consumer exposure to cosmetics is enormous."

So if you think it's time for Congress to discontinue its laissez-faire attitude that results in cosmetic trick-or-treat for consumers, experience has shown that election years are the very best time to nudge your legislators. Witness the Eagleton bill, which gave the senator a head start on his run for re-election with television appearances on the news programs and talk shows when he introduced his cosmetic safety bill that eventually died after his election.

The moral is that a nudge before election deserves two after election.

— 3 —
When Is a Cosmetic a Drug...
and a Drug a Cosmetic?

The drug versus cosmetic question can be as
baffling to our field investigators as it may be to
representatives of the cosmetic industry.
—Heinz J. Eiermann, Director,
Division of Cosmetics Technology

When is a deodorant an antiperspirant? When does
a cosmetic become a drug? If a cream is a cosmetic, how come
it's a drug? Suntan lotions or sunscreens—which are the
drugs? Cinnamon-flavored toothpicks are *cosmetics*?

Ambiguity is the name of the game. The game is always
played in courts where time is never called, errors never
counted, penalties never assessed; and the taxpaying consumers are the ultimate, definitive, habitual losers footing the bill
and bearing the bruises.

Take a category most consumers don't even know
exists—that of drug "cosmetics." How does one explain that an
underarm deodorant can contain the same ingredients as one that
calls itself an "antiperspirant" and be classified as a cosmetic
requiring no testing for safety or efficacy? If it is labeled as an

"antiperspirant," it becomes a drug and subject to the drug regulations that require proof of safety and effectiveness, full directions for use, warnings against misuse, and tighter manufacturing controls.

The metamorphosis occurs with a change of claims. The deodorant claims only to protect against odor; the antiperspirant claims to protect against wetness—or to change a bodily function, which the FDA claims makes it a drug. Some underarm products straddle both categories. The Speed Stick by Mennen, for instance, calls itself a "SUPER DRY ANTIPERSPIRANT deodorant" and promises "Long lasting protection against odor and wetness."

As FDA's Heinz Eiermann explained it, the FD&C Act defines cosmetics as articles intended to be applied to the human body for cleansing, beautifying, promoting attractiveness, or altering the appearance. Drugs are defined as articles intended to cure, mitigate, treat, or prevent disease and articles intended to affect the structure or any function of the body.

Since the two categories are not mutually exclusive, articles intended to cleanse, beautify, or promote attractiveness as well as treat or prevent disease or otherwise affect the structure or any function of the human body are both drugs and cosmetics and must comply with the regulatory requirements of both categories.

Sometimes an active ingredient such as estrogenic hormones can change a cream or lotion from a cosmetic into a drug. Hormone drug cosmetics, however, have thus far escaped proving themselves to be effective drugs, having been on the market before the 1962 Kefauver-Harris Amendments to the FD&C Act required "substantial evidence" of effectiveness of a new drug for the uses, indications, and claims in the labeling.

When it comes to categorizing suntan and sunscreen products, even the FDA seems confused. In 1940, the agency took the position that articles that refer in labeling to sunburn are *drugs,* and articles that are represented exclusively for the production of a tan are regarded as *cosmetics.*

Accordingly, a product containing a sunscreening agent and claiming to prevent sunburn is a *drug,* and a product not containing a sunscreening agent and claiming that it helps promote an even tan is a *cosmetic.*

But what about the sunscreen-containing product that claims to help promote an even tan and is silent about the sunscreening effect? In 1976, the FDA said it had moved away from judging the category by its label and "has concluded that a product containing a sunscreen ingredient. . . , even when labeled solely as a tanning aid, is both intended and understood to be a preventative of sunburn, and is therefore a *drug.*"

However, since the agency had not yet publicly revoked the old category-by-label theory, it said it would continue to treat the suntan and sunscreen products as it had in the past.

In 1978, an FDA-appointed advisory panel recommended that "regardless of claims, products intended to be used for prevention of sunburn or any similar condition should be regarded as *drugs.*"

And so the FDA dutifully published its proposed rule to treat the sunscreens and the suntan-sunscreens as drugs; but until it becomes a regulation, the agency will continue to separate the drugs from the cosmetics according to labeling even though the ingredients may be the same. And, of course, the cosmetic industry, represented by its Washington organizations, lobbyists, and lawyers, will fight the proposed rule in and out of the courts—and will win time and time and time . . .

Meanwhile, back on Jekyll Island, Georgia, once a haven for the Rockefellers and similar folk, Heinz Eiermann was telling a meeting of cosmetic chemists: "The drug versus cosmetic question can be as baffling to our field investigators as it may be to representatives of the cosmetic industry. An inspector is often faced with the decision whether to examine a product as a drug or as a cosmetic and, accordingly, inspect a manufacturing plant as a drug establishment or as one manufacturing cosmetics. In our current Compliance Program Guidance Manual, we advise our inspectors to consider a product declaring an active ingredient to be a drug. If the ingredient declaration does not identify an active ingredient, the inspector is to treat the product as a cosmetic. Of course, depending on other label statements, that product could also be a misbranded drug."

That was in March 1982—only *four* years since the FDA published its proposal back in D.C. to make all suntan and sunscreen products drugs, regardless of labels—and *four* years since its advisory panel handed in its report after mulling over the problem for three years—and *six* years since the FDA changed its mind and decided that all those products were drugs after all.

The taxpaying consumers who had footed the bill for Mr. Eiermann's excursion to Jekyll Island to tell the cosmetic chemists what they already knew, and who were buying the drug cosmetics or the cosmetic cosmetics that had made it possible for the cosmetic chemists to be employed and to be sent to Jekyll Island for their meeting by their benevolent employers, were not even mentioned in the now-you-see-it-now-you-don't game that supposedly was being played for *their* benefit.

The cinnamon-flavored toothpicks? The FDA claimed those were cosmetics and, for years, seized batch after batch for reasons best forgotten.

QUESTIONS AND ANSWERS

What is the main difference in a cosmetic product that is classified as a cosmetic or as a drug?

In intent, a drug-cosmetic claims to affect the structure or a function of the body. For instance, any product that would claim to grow hair on a bald head would classify as a drug even though it might call itself a pomade, which ordinarily would be considered to be a cosmetic for grooming the hair.

In regulation, the drug-cosmetic would have to adhere to the stricter drug regulations that would include registration, premarket testing to prove safety and efficacy, as well as being subject to stricter manufacturing practices and inspection—all of which a product classified as a cosmetic escapes.

Suntan and sunscreen products now have numbers on their labels. How do I choose the right number for me?

The FDA had an advisory panel work on this. As a result, the following categories were established with the recommended Sun Protection Factor (SPF) numbers.

Pick the number that most closely fits your requirements, but don't overdo your exposure to sun regardless of your choice.

MINIMAL SUN PROTECTION: SPF 2 to 4. Least protection, but permit suntanning.

MODERATE SUN PROTECTION: SPF 4 and 5. Moderate protection from sunburning, but permit some suntanning.

EXTRA SUN PROTECTION: SPF 6 and 7. Extra protection from sunburning, and permit limited suntanning.

MAXIMAL SUN PROTECTION: SPF 8 through 14. Maximal protection from sunburning, and permit little or no suntanning.

ULTRA SUN PROTECTION: SPF 15 or greater. Most protection from sunburning, and permit no suntanning.

— 4 —
The Fragrant Allergen

Ingredients which FDA accepts as "trade
secrets" and the ingredients of flavors and
fragrances need not be specifically declared.
—Food and Drug Administration

Every other person is allergic to something. It has
been estimated that 50 percent of the population is subject to
allergic reactions.

Other people's allergies have been extremely profitable
for the cosmetic industry. It has both made and saved money
from allergies, real and alleged.

While it may be true that there has yet to be a cata-
strophic epidemic of consumers falling dead because of a cosmetic, there have been blindings, deaths, multiple injuries to
eyes, nails, skin, and scalp, damage and loss of hair, burns, skin
discolorations, and evidence of systemic changes and disease.

Although the industry repeatedly blames personal and
individual allergy and/or misuse in defending charges of injuries and untoward reactions, court trials and investigations
have shown that many of the products involved had not been

sufficiently tested for otherwise predictably unsafe ingredients before being marketed.

A clause in Section 740.10 of the Food, Drug, and Cosmetic Act titled **"Labeling of cosmetic products for which adequate substantiation of safety has not been obtained,"** states: "Each ingredient used in a cosmetic product and each finished cosmetic product shall be adequately substantiated for safety prior to marketing. Any such ingredient or product whose safety is not adequately substantiated prior to marketing is misbranded unless it contains the following conspicuous statement on the principal display panel: *Warning*—The safety of this product has not been determined."

Since the FDA cannot and does not require manufacturers to test any cosmetic ingredient, except color, or any product classified as a cosmetic, Section 740.10 asks manufacturers for a public confession to be made in a "conspicuous statement on the principal display panel."

Having examined thousands of cosmetic packages, from the elite to the scruffy, and not found a single label warning me that the safety of the product had not been determined, I now plan to follow Alice through the looking glass into Wonderland, where I expect to find the FDA along with the Easter bunny.

Furthermore, I've yet to hear of any manufacturer being charged with marketing a misbranded cosmetic because the safety of an ingredient or a product was determined not to have been adequately substantiated prior to marketing. Nor have I heard of any punitive action taken by the FDA as a result of Section 740.10.

Meanwhile, the key men of the skeleton staff allotted to cosmetics, with the entire cosmetic program budgeted at less than two and a half million dollars and at much less than one percent of the FDA annual budget, dissipate time and funds in traveling the industry convention circuit in and out of the country with speeches that reiterate the sins of the industry to the industry. In recent years, the circuit has stretched from Santiago, Chile, in October to Boca Raton, Florida, in February and March.

The principals rarely, if ever, are found at a consumer's meeting in Des Moines in January or in Newark in August. Most likely, consumers will hear the local "consumer affairs officer" in a recital of the "FDA's role in cosmetic protection for the consumer." Most likely, no mention will be made of AETT, 6-MC, nitrosamines, chloroform, vinyl chloride, and 1,4-dioxane, all of which had the potential of being detrimental to the health of unprotected consumers, and which Deputy Director John A. Wenninger, of the FDA's Division of Cosmetics Technology, discussed in his speech to industry members attending an international symposium in New York in September.

The following month, Heinz J. Eiermann, director of the same division, traveled to Chile to repeat the litany to a Latin American convention, adding formaldehyde, vitamin E, methylmethacrylate, pathogenic microorganisms, and nonpermitted color additives, all of which had the potential to cause harm when found in cosmetics used by unprotected consumers.

In another year, the beginning of March found FDA Commissioner Arthur Hull Hayes, Jr., going over the same ground in Boca Raton at The Cosmetics, Toiletry and Fragrance Association's convention. He threw in hexachlorophene, which, indeed, had caused harm to unprotected consumers.

And yet no mention was made of any action that might have resulted from Section 740.10, although, apparently, none of the products with the offending ingredients carried the prescribed "Warning—The safety of this product has not been determined."

While ingredient listing, begun in 1977, has helped those who know to which ingredient they are allergic, the absence of fragrance and flavor identification continues to cause problems. Even those who are fairly free from allergies can become sensitized and react from photosensitizing fragrance ingredients. They may then find themselves with permanent dark or brown patches of skin as a result of the sun's effect on the fragrance ingredient.

There probably wasn't a single representative from the fragrance industry to whom John Wenninger was speaking who was not aware of 6-MC (6-methylcoumarin). Consumers throughout the nation, however, might have been interested to know that 6-MC was a fragrance ingredient that had been added to suntan and sunscreen products, and then was found to have caused severe reactions when exposed to the sun.

Mr. Wenninger described it as a potent photocontact allergen (a photosensitizer).

According to the deputy director: "One major concern we had with continued use of 6-MC in suntan products was the possible induction of sensitization in a wide segment of the population not already allergic to the substance. In addition, the adverse reactions related to 6-MC in some products were not the usual transitory skin effects often associated with cosmetic allergic relations. Some reports described blistering of the skin and systemic effects that in some cases required hospitalization of the affected person. A recall of such products was the best course of action we could follow to prevent further consumer exposure to the harmful effect of 6-MC."

He might have added that the FDA explained that the reaction could lead to a chronic condition in which a sensitized person can have a skin reaction simply by being exposed to sunlight. All this from perfume added to sunscreens that did nothing to improve their efficacy.

Assumptions can be dangerous, but in this instance it would be safe to assume the people who bought sunscreens bought them so they *could* expose themselves to the sun more safely than otherwise. In fact, many consumers may have been prompted to buy sunscreens after hearing or reading the highly publicized FDA report from its own appointed, tax-funded expert advisory committee. In an eight-page publicity release, issued just months before December 5, 1978, when the FDA announced that it was asking manufacturers to eliminate 6-MC from their suntan and sunscreen products, consumers were advised that "proper use of sunscreen products to prevent sunburn may protect against premature aging of the skin and possibly skin cancer." It also would be safe to assume that there was great cheering from the producers of sunscreens at this free official promotional bonanza.

Mr. Wenninger told his audience that the FDA alerted the industry to the problem and "requested" that the industry remove 6-MC from their products. Left unsaid was the report that, for a number of years, the FDA had been notified by Plough, a major manufacturer of sunscreens including Coppertone, Lipkote, and Tropical Blend, that it had received numerous consumer complaints about reactions suffered after using some of Plough's products. As a result, Plough had isolated the fragrance ingredient as a source of the problem and had halted shipments of products containing 6-MC.

In the December 1978–January 1979 *FDA Consumer,* the agency's own magazine, FDA reported that Plough had not shipped any products with 6-MC for "about a year." However, "FDA does not know what other suntan preparations or other drug or cosmetic products contain 6-methylcoumarin. The Food, Drug, and Cosmetic Act does not require manufacturers to tell the Agency the ingredients in its fragrances, and fragrance ingredients do not have to be listed on the label.

FDA now is testing suntan products on the market to determine whether they contain this fragrance ingredient."

The FDA sent telegrams to those sunscreen manufacturers and fragrance suppliers *known to it* to discontinue using
6-MC, to recall any products containing the ingredient, and to
identify the products with 6-MC so that the public could be informed. Although there is a voluntary registration program,
cosmetic manufacturers are not required to register with the
FDA, so that not even the FDA could contact many companies
who see no advantage to confessing they exist.

For those reached by the FDA, the reply date was set
for December 14, 1978, but months passed without further
word to potential consumers.

Plough wasn't alone in receiving complaints. FDA admitted that it had received "numerous reports" from injured
consumers "over the past few years," and Mr. Wenninger cited
"documented case histories of consumer adverse reactions to
products containing 6-MC." There was no explanation, however, as to why it had taken the agency so long to make its announcement while encouraging the public to slather on more
and more sunscreens.

Even more puzzling was FDA's disclosure in December 1978 that Plough had not only halted shipment of 6-
MC-containing sunscreens, but also had assured the agency
that, although its Tropical Blend previously had contained 6-
MC, it had been reformulated. Yet, on February 7, 1979, the
FDA announced that Plough had recalled certain lots of its
Tropical Blend Dark Tanning Oil and Lotion on September 22,
1978. The announcement came almost five months after Plough
said it had sent its salesmen out to recall the lotion and oil—
and about a year and nine months after Plough said it had
stopped shipment. The FDA also reported that the firm had in-
itiated an ongoing recall and "that very little remains on the
market."

Five days after the FDA announcement, Plough issued its own press release protesting the FDA recall listing, calling it "unwarranted" and claiming that Plough had not agreed to the action.

In December 1978, the FDA said it would "consider the need for further regulatory action after evaluating all information" and that it would propose a regulation to ban 6-MC in all cosmetic products and drugs intended for use on the skin. Plough was reported to have "totally" supported the proposed ban on 6-MC—and possibly also coumarin, which had been in Lipkote but had since been eliminated.

Almost ten months later Deputy Director Wenninger said the FDA was "planning to publish regulations which will prohibit the use of 6-MC . . . in cosmetics and topical drugs."

The industry successfully deflected the regulations by assuring the FDA that it had voluntarily discontinued the use of 6-MC.

During the sparring between the FDA and Plough, as well as the rest of the industry, there was no suggestion that the better solution to the "guess which sunscreen has the not-so-good-for-you ingredient" might be the listing of fragrance ingredients on the label.

Mr. Wenninger did remark on "the traditional secrecy which surrounds the composition of fragrance preparations" during his speech to the industry.

According to the Cosmetics Division deputy director: "The ingredients of specific fragrances are unknown to the public, FDA and most cosmetic firms who incorporate them into their products. Requiring the listing of fragrance ingredients has been suggested in the past but not adopted by FDA because of the trade secret issues raised and the complexity of fragrance formulations."

A suffering consumer might have pointed out that sunscreens are not considered by the public to be "fragrance formulations." Since fragrance adds nothing to the efficacy of a sunscreen, why would consumers, made even more cautious about exposing themselves to the sun by a supposedly protective agency, want to expose themselves to a hidden risk of injury because some chemist decided the sunscreen should smell one way or another?

After all, the expert panel, paid with tax dollars, *did* recommend that all sunscreen products include the message: **"Overexposure to the sun may lead to premature aging of the skin and skin cancer. The liberal and regular use of this product may reduce the chance of premature aging of the skin and skin cancer."**

If there's room on a label for that message, surely room could be found for fragrance ingredients that need not be complex and might, indeed, be eliminated. Maybe now that we know that 6-MC carries a risk, it would help to know which sunscreen or any other cosmetic may still have it. If the chemist is paid for giving us his choice, shouldn't the potential consumers who are paying be given their choice?

QUESTIONS AND ANSWERS

When there is a recall of a cosmetic that has been found to be hazardous or, for some reason, may pose a risk to the user, what is done to retrieve the cosmetic from someone who may have bought it before the stores took it off the shelves?

Unless the buyer is aware of the recall and refrains from using the product, very little, if anything, is done to attempt to call the product back from the consumer who may have bought it. Usually nothing is done, and the consumers are lucky if they're informed through the public media that there is something wrong with the cosmetic.

In the case of the suntan oil and lotion with 6-MC,

which both the company and the FDA knew might cause problems if the products were used in the sun, as intended, the products remained in the market for years without potential buyers and users being warned of the risk.

When the FDA issues a warning or announces a recall, is it automatically reported in the newspapers and on television and radio?

Not always. It's up to the individual newspaper or radio or television station.

Suppose I find that I have a cosmetic that has been recalled from the stores or has been reported as having a problem, what should I do with the cosmetic?

Don't use it. The cosmetic company would prefer that you throw it away. I wouldn't. I'd take it back to where I bought it. I'd suggest that the product be returned to the manufacturer and ask for a refund or an exchange for another product.

If the merchant is unwilling to accommodate you, send the product back to the cosmetic company and ask for a refund.

Even though I know a product has been recalled, I still see it being sold. Aren't recalls enforced?

Hardly. Most recalls are voluntary, and the FDA seems to take a grateful posture even when a cosmetic has been proven to be injurious and may have injured. For a regulatory agency, the FDA often seems to lack strength when it comes to dealing with the cosmetic industry.

In case some of the Tropical Blend sunscreens are still around—or maybe in my medicine cabinet left over from earlier summers—which lots were picked up by Plough?

The lots reported as being recalled were: Tropical Blend Dark Tanning Lotion, in 8-fluid-ounce containers and

1/2-fluid-ounce containers; all three-digit lot numbers; and all five-digit lot numbers prior to but not including 7P392. Also: Tropical Blend Dark Tanning Oil in 8-fluid-ounce containers; all three-digit numbers; and all five-digit lot numbers prior to but not including 7P387.

— 5 —
Read Any Good Labels Lately?

The label on each package of a cosmetic shall
bear a declaration of the name of each ingredient
in descending order of predominance, except that
fragrance or flavor may be listed as fragrance or
flavor.
—Code of Federal Regulations

Did you know that, until 1977, you could read a label and find out what was stuffing your mattress or the fiber content of your sheets and clothing, but not what was in the toothpaste you put in your mouth? Any product classified as a cosmetic was exempted from ingredient disclosure—not only on labels, but to physicians and government officials as well. No cosmetic ingredient was required to be disclosed even when a cosmetic or a cosmetic ingredient was suspected of having caused injury, illness, or death.

After multiple delays obtained by the cosmetic industry, hundreds of thousands of cosmetic products are now required to list their ingredients on all packages except those intended for professional use. It's no secret that consumer pressure forced the Food and Drug Administration to issue

mandatory ingredient listing regulations after voluntary ingredient listing failed miserably. The regulations were promulgated under the 1966 Fair Packaging and Labeling Act, which
empowered the Secretary of the Department of Health, Education and Welfare, FDA's umbrella department, to do so "to
prevent deception or to facilitate value comparison" or both.
The ingredients were to be listed by their common names, if
possible, and in the order of decreasing predominance without
disclosing "trade secrets."

There are exemptions. For instance: All ingredients are
required to be listed except *flavors and fragrances.* The exemption was won by the cosmetic industry with a plea that the
components of fragrances, in particular, were too complex and
too numerous to list. Perhaps overlooked was the fact that the
identical plea had been used to forestall the listing of colors
and of *any* and *all* ingredients.

Ironically, the perfumes used in cosmetics have been
consistently implicated in causing allergic reactions and have
hastened the trend toward so-called hypo-allergenic cosmetics—many of which simply omit perfume.

Although fragrance and flavors contribute nothing to
the efficacy of a cosmetic, they can be added without any requirement for testing or disclosure of any kind. As the law
stands, none of the ingredients used in a cosmetic product, except color (which must be listed), is required to be tested for
purity, safety, toxicity, hazards, or anything else.

Color additives, which have come under the most scru-
tiny, must be tested and certified before they can legally be
added to a cosmetic—a regulation inherited from the colors
also used in food and drugs. However, except for now having
to list ingredients, hair dyes, the most dangerous of colors, are
entirely exempted from the meager controls of other cosmetics.

Although hair dyes did not escape the labeling regulations, permanent coal-tar hair dyes still enjoy complete ex-

emption from the 1938 Food, Drug, and Cosmetic Act. The initial exemption was won by the industry because it claimed that it could not make permanent hair dyes without the admittedly dangerous coal-tar dyes.

The exemption was granted with the provision that packages bear the warning: "CAUTION: This product contains ingredients which may cause skin irritations on certain individuals and a preliminary patch test according to accompanying directions should first be made. This product should not be used for dyeing the eyelashes or eyebrows; to do so may cause blindness."

However, since many women and men have their hair dyed in beauty and barber shops, many women and men do not see the package with its warning and remain unaware that the patch test was intended to precede *every* hair dyeing to avoid the possible severe allergic reactions.

And although hair dyes were caught in the ingredient-labeling net and their unsafe as well as innocuous ingredients must be listed on packages sold over the counter to consumers, the professional packages sold to barbers and beauticians remain legally without the ingredients listed. Neither the operator nor the customer, therefore, knows for sure whether the latest ingredient to be found to be a potent carcinogen is in the hair dye being used.

QUESTIONS AND ANSWERS

I can't understand the chemical names on the labels. Where can I find out what they mean?

Since common chemical names are to be used whenever possible, most of the chemical names are names of chemicals that can be looked up in a chemical dictionary or *The Merck Index* and *The Physician's Desk Reference*, both of which will give possible side effects or reactions. Try your local library for the books.

If you are unable to find the chemicals listed in those reference books, try the latest *CTFA Cosmetic Ingredient Dictionary*, compiled by The Cosmetic, Toiletry and Fragrance Association, which may be available in specialized libraries.

If you still need more information, you might try writing to the cosmetic company and/or to The Cosmetic, Toiletry and Fragrance Association, Inc., 1110 Vermont Ave., N.W., Suite 800, Washington, D.C. 20005, as well as to the Director, Division of Cosmetics Technology, Food and Drug Administration, 200 C Street, S.W., Washington, D.C. 20204.

Of what value is the listing of ingredients?

The obvious value, especially to the allergic consumer, is being able to avoid offending allergens in a product before buying and using it.

Less obvious is the sanitizing effect of having to list an ingredient that is known to have caused harm or may be capable of causing harm. An example is that of 2,4-toluenediamine, or 2,4-TDA, which had been in a number of hair dyes when it was revealed as having caused cancerous growths and liver cancer in animal research dating back to 1949. Only when this was belatedly reported in the news was the ingredient hurriedly removed from many of the new batches of hair dyes. The old packages with the revealed ingredient were not recalled, however, and remained on the store shelves to be carried away by unaware buyers. The aware buyers could read the labels and choose the packages without 2,4-TDA.

Some supermarkets have generic products that cost less than advertised brands. Are there generic cosmetics?

Staple cosmetic products such as toothpaste and shampoo can be found in the generic sections of supermarkets.

However, the generic equivalent of other cosmetics can be found as "private label" cosmetics. These cosmetics may be made by some of the same manufacturers who make the big-name cosmetics. The labels, minus the advertising hoopla, usually are of the store selling the cosmetics.

In reading the labels on so many of the cosmetics, I see that water is the first ingredient used. Does this mean that, when I pay $5 or more, I'm buying mostly water?

Yes. That is one reason why the industry was reluctant to list its ingredients in the order of predominance. One segment of the industry continued to fight, even after the regulation was passed, to list the ingredients alphabetically. In this way, even sharp consumers, such as you, might not realize that many, if not most, cosmetics are predominantly water—and, apparently, very expensive water.

I notice that many of the creams contain pretty much the same ingredients, yet some are priced at a fraction of others. In fact, I saw the same ingredients on a cream that was priced at $1 and on another that was priced at $20 an ounce. Why the difference in price?

I asked a leading cosmetic merchandiser the same question. His answer was that the difference was in what he called "psychological pricing." Prospective buyers might be tempted to believe that a $20 cream must be twenty times better than a $1 cream, and a $60 "miracle" cream at least three times better than the $20 cream. According to the merchandiser, whose store sold all three, cosmetic companies are more than willing to accommodate the believers by offering them $20 or $60 worth of hope. The basic ingredients may be similar or identical in all the creams. The more expensive creams may have a flick of exotic or "scientific-miracle" ingredient promoted with glowing promises and psychologically priced accordingly. The greatest benefit, according to the merchandiser, is to the manufacturer, distributor, retailer, and commission-paid salespeople. Logically, many more $1 cream sales would have to be made to equal the one-time sale and profit of the $20 or $60 cream.

Given a choice of a cosmetic with a long list of ingredients and a similar cosmetic with fewer ingredients, which would you recommend buying?

If the cosmetic is one that doesn't depend on a blending of pigments to attain a particular shade of color, I'd buy the one with the fewer ingredients. Since nothing but color needs to be tested, I'd rather chance a few than many ingredients even though, until Congress and the FDA mandate premarket testing, it's still trick-or-treat for consumers.

I was shocked to find that, although there are signs in supermarkets warning that saccharin has been found to cause cancer in animals, all the popular and generic brands of toothpaste contain saccharin. Why is this being forced upon those of us who prefer to avoid saccharin?

Leading toothpaste manufacturers were asked this question. The answer given was that saccharin was put into toothpaste to sweeten it for children. There was no answer to the question of who decided that toothpaste *should* be sweet so that children, thereafter, would expect sweet toothpaste.

My suggestion to one company that adults be given a choice of saccharin and nonsaccharin toothpaste was followed by an advertising campaign about an "adult" toothpaste. The "adult" toothpaste, however, still contained saccharin.

If you and others would direct your disapproval of saccharin in toothpaste to the manufacturers and suggest that discerning and buying adults be given a choice, some company is bound to take notice and smell a profit.

I notice that, although formaldehyde is known to be bad news and can cause painful problems with nails, just about every nail polish I've seen has it listed as an ingredient. Is it a necessary ingredient for all nail polish?

Apparently not. Hypo-allergenic lines omit formaldehyde. Also, nonformaldehyde nail products are fairly common in Egypt, Israel, and other countries. Letters to cosmetic company executives pointing out your preference might prove influential. At least they'll now know that potential buyers do read labels even though many of them have insisted that no one would read the ingredients if they listed them.

— 6 —
Scents and Non-Scents

No ingredient may be designated as fragrance or
flavor unless it is within the meaning of such term
as commonly understood by consumers.
—FDA Designation of Ingredients

Until recent years, the skin was thought to be an almost impenetrable barrier. Research has shown that this was a mistaken assumption.

In 1978, Dr. Joseph Faucher of Union Carbide Corporation, a major supplier of chemicals used in cosmetics, chided the cosmetic industry for often ignoring or denying that topically applied preparations could actually go into the human hair and skin. He suggested that economic and psychological reasons might account for the attitude.

Dr. Faucher said he was convinced that topically applied preparations went beyond the surface when his experiments showed that shampoo left on the scalp for a minute resulted in "a fair amount going into the scalp." Further study was needed, he told his audience of cosmetic chemists, adding

34

that more was known of calf hair and skin than of human hair and skin.

During the 1983 convention of the Cosmetic, Toiletry and Fragrance Association, the trade association whose active members market about 90 percent of the cosmetic products sold in the United States, FDA Commissioner Arthur Hull Hayes, Jr., elaborated on the new awareness of skin penetration.

According to Dr. Hayes: "Since passage of the FD&C Act, scientists have learned that there is, next to ingestion and inhalation, a third route of exposure of man to chemicals. Though absorption of a substance through the skin is usually less than through intestinal or lung tissue, the twenty square feet of skin surface nevertheless offer much opportunity for exposure and systemic harm. This I know from firsthand experience as a physician. The systemic effects from topical exposure to hexachlorophene and AETT (acetylethyl tetramethyl tetralin), for example, have taught us that application of biologically active substances to the skin is not without risk and that any assessment of the risk of man's exposure to a material must also take into consideration exposure to the skin."

In the case of hexachlorophene (HCP), it took a long time before the lesson got through to the FDA. For decades, hexachlorophene was trumpeted as the "plus" ingredient in cosmetics that ranged from baby products to makeup. At a time when no cosmetic ingredient needed to be disclosed, the industry found it commercially feasible to advertise it as a good-for-you additive that killed nasty germs.

Although pediatricians advise the avoidance of medicated toiletries for infants and children in families with a history of allergies, even with the dethroning of hexachlorophene, it remains difficult to find baby products that do not include unwarranted and unnecessary medication.

While hexachlorophene was the ubiquitous king, the FDA estimated that as much as 30 percent of all cosmetics on the market contained HCP. For decades, cosmetic products for the entire family carried the HCP message on its label. Every member of the family was likely to be hexachlorophened twenty-four hours a day. In addition to the baby washes, lotions, creams, cleansers, and talcum powder, the family collection might have included hexachlorophened toothpaste, mouthwash, deodorant, antiperspirant, talc, the whole range of preshave, shave, and postshave products, all kinds of creams, lotions, makeup, and hair products, and the then popular "intimate sprays."

From the beginning, *The Merck Index of Chemicals and Drugs* warned that the disinfectant could cause sensitivity reactions. In 1964, medical reports implicated HCP in a cross-sensitizing link that resulted in photodermatitis, or adverse skin reactions triggered by exposure to sunlight. These were followed by a succession of studies, surveys, and tests, including some by the FDA.

Further reports showed that deaths had occurred after burn patients had been treated with HCP preparations. Fed to rats, the germicide caused brain damage. Tested on human beings, hexachlorophene was absorbed through the skin and was found in measurable quantities in the blood. When it was used on babies, some suffered convulsions.

Still, in April 1971, the FDA announced it planned no regulatory action. In May, the American Academy of Pediatrics' Committee on Environmental Hazards warned parents not to allow children to use oral preparations containing HCP, such as toothpaste and mouthwash. A child had died after swallowing a few ounces of a 3-percent hexachlorophene solution.

In June, to answer the numerous inquiries it was receiving, the FDA prepared an "updated response statement." In part, it read:

> Hexachlorophene as an active ingredient in various formulations was cleared for safety through the new drug procedure early in the history of the 1938 Food, Drug, and Cosmetic Act. More recent experience has indicated that in certain circumstances toxic amounts can be absorbed. Studies by FDA toxicologists and other FDA scientists, as well as outside investigators are currently under way to extend our knowledge of hexachlorophene under various conditions of use.

Continuing FDA tests found that hexachlorophene "is absorbed and blood levels can be detected in the normal population." In animals, the FDA reported, "High levels produced brain damage and convulsions."

On September 25, 1972, *The Wall Street Journal* reported "new evidence of potential dangers—including a University of Washington study that found on a preliminary basis that brain damage occurred among newborn infants who had been routinely washed with hexachlorophene solutions. University experts examined at autopsy 204 infants, some premature, who had died from other causes, but had been washed with hexachlorophene to prevent infection."

Dr. Ellsworth Elvord, Jr., professor of pathology at the University of Washington, also had reported to the FDA that he had found a definite correlation between three or more documented exposures to HCP and lesions in the brain stem. But it took the news that thirty to forty babies in France had died after being dusted with talcum powder that contained too much HCP to rouse the FDA into action.

Only then did the FDA attempt to rid the market of HCP in vigorously advertised, casually used products with a recall. HCP was then restricted to prescriptive drugs to be used "when, in the judgment of the physician, the risk of toxicity is outweighed by its effectiveness in controlling infection."

With AETT (acetyl ethyl tetramethyl tetralin), FDA found another horror story.

To escape possible sensitization or allergic reactions to fragrance, many consumers have turned to cosmetics labeled "unscented." Unrealized is the fact that "unscented" does not mean *without fragrance ingredients.*

Some "unscented" label packages now list "masking fragrance," but since fragrance ingredients do not have to be identified—they're not.

AETT was primarily used as a fixative or masking ingredient. It was also a fragrance oil, and it would have been better for everyone if it had been listed.

Used for twenty-two years in everyday staples such as soap, aftershave, and deodorants, AETT was found to have triggered a series of systemic changes, not the least of which was nerve damage. AETT proved that cosmetics could not *only* carry risks of allergic reactions for the allergic, but could carry risks to the general public through the skin and respiratory channels.

Chilling laboratory test reports and related material, obtained through the Freedom of Information Act, traced the questioning of AETT back to July 1975 when Avon toxicologists, through routine testing, found that AETT "produced in rats a blue color of most internal organs, including the brain."

Previous AETT tests using rabbits did not turn the animals' insides blue. With rats, however, AETT oxidized, binding with tissue components. The blue color was detectable in rats "within a short period of time." Later tests show that rabbits' insides also turned blue.

Avon's concern increased when a six-month study with AETT "produced not only the blue coloration of tissues but also produced brain and spinal cord vacuolization . . . [and] confirmed the presence of neurotoxicity." At the time, Avon was marketing a number of cosmetics with AETT, ranging from its DemiStick solid fragrance with .95 percent AETT and Cream Sachet with .45 percent, to its Skin Softener with .033 percent and Men's Cologne with .008 percent.

As the tests and studies continued, the discoveries became more and more startling. A single topical application of an AETT compound produced the blue color in rats and was observed seven days after the application. Inhalation of an AETT-containing aerosol was enough to turn the rat's insides blue.

Signs of toxicity were "hyperactivity, tremors, death; peculiar blue coloration of internal organs including brain and spinal cord. Hyperexcitability on subacute exposure."

Cumulative signs of toxicity included "hyperexcitability, incoordination, hunched back, weight loss, tremors, and unresponsiveness."

The tests extended into late 1977 with Givaudan, one of the two major suppliers of AETT, joining Avon in the various studies. On October 17, 1977, Arthur D. Little, Inc., submitted a 57-page report on tests begun for Givaudan in an attempt to find an explanation for the blue-color "phenomenon."

According to the report, "The ultimate objective was to have in hand data which would permit a better estimate of this (blue color) phenomenon in humans."

The studies failed to explain the phenomenon. However, the clinically detailed laboratory report, replete with photographs of dissected rats, dispelled any remaining doubt that the "phenomenon" indicated more than a coloring trick. Prominent among the toxic symptons were weight loss, gastrointestinal tract abnormality, and death.

Female rats were more vulnerable to the "fragrance" when it was given in doses of 50 milligrams per kilogram. Death was total among the female rats; but AETT also claimed 33.3 percent of the males.

More bad news came in October 1977. In a neuropathological evaluation of rats after eleven weeks of treatment, Dr. Peter S. Spencer of the Albert Einstein College of Medicine reported "widespread neuropathological damage ... [confirmation of] the potential of AETT as a neurotoxin. Widespread vacuolization of the spinal cord and cerebellar area ... along with demyelination of peripheral nerves."

Simply, in these and later studies, Dr. Spencer effectively proved that AETT, tested on rats, was disrupting the spinal cord, brain, and nerve sheaths.

On November 4, 1977, Dr. Donald Opdyke, president of the Research Institute for Fragrance Materials (RIFM), requested a meeting with the FDA to inform the agency of the animal-testing results of AETT.

On November 7, RIFM advised its members that experiments carried out in "the last three years" showed AETT to have "a potential for producing neurotoxic effects and/or generalized tissue discoloration in several species of laboratory animals. Despite the absence of reported effects of this sort in man, prudence would dictate the avoidance of this material in fragrance compounds."

No mention was made of Givaudan's "human percutaneous study designed to measure skin penetration, absorption and excretion of topically applied" AETT.

In Givaudan's report to the FDA, the company explained that with the first report of toxicity caused by AETT, which it manufactured, "it became more urgent to find the significance of these results in regard to human exposure." Preliminary results of the human percutaneous tests confirmed that the chemical was absorbed through the skin and found in the urine.

While the tests were in progress, Avon definitely established that AETT produced serious nerve damage, and it was decided to submit the available data to the RIFM panel of experts for evaluation. On the panel's recommendation, "Givaudan ceased manufacture of fragrances containing AETT. It is our thinking now to try to continue the study in humans to elucidate the mechanism of excretion and metabolism and thus make possible a valid assessment of the animal data."

Asked whether Givaudan had continued its tests, Dr. Julian Dorsky, Givaudan's vice-president of research and development, said, "No, it became apparent in the course of our tests that this was not a compound to be defended."

A day before industry representatives met with members of the FDA, RIFM's expert panel agreed to notify members to cease using AETT in their products, but felt that "no recall of products containing AETT was deemed necessary."

Marketed under two trade names—Versalide Extra by Givaudan in the United States and Switzerland, and Musk 36A by UOP Chemical in the United States—AETT is also known as "polycyclic musk" and "musk tetralin." In recent years, a Japanese company also became a supplier of AETT. An estimated .75 million pounds of AETT annually found its way into a wide variety of consumer products, from soaps and detergents to lotions, creams, sachets, perfumes, colognes, aftershaves, antiperspirant ... and "unscented" deodorants and hairsprays.

A few antiperspirants, which are classified as drugs, listed their brand of AETT in their ingredient labeling. Deodorants, which are classified as cosmetics, are not required to list fragrances, and—scented or unscented—the deodorants escaped listing the neurotoxin as it sailed under the industry-protective "fragrance" banner.

The disclosure that AETT had been used as a *masking agent* to overcome less fragrant ingredients in cosmetics labeled as "unscented" raised questions that remain unanswered. If AETT—or any other ingredient, be it a fragrance component or otherwise—has been used for purposes other than to add fragrance, can or should it escape listing as a fragrance ingredient?

FDA's own "Designation of ingredients" clause 701.3 states: "No ingredient may be designated as fragrance or flavor unless it is within the meaning of such term as commonly understood by consumers."

The *CTFA Labeling Manual* advises that, according to the FDA, "The term 'fragrance' means any natural or synthetic substance or substances used solely to impart an odor to a cosmetic product."

The industry manual warns, "A manufacturer must exercise sound judgement in deciding when use of the terms 'flavor' or 'fragrance' is appropriate ... FDA could charge that an ill-supported designation of an ingredient as a 'flavor' or 'fragrance' was adopted as a guise to avoid chemical declaration of an ingredient."

It is probable that a poll of consumers would find that the overwhelming majority would interpret "unscented" to mean exactly that.

In the case of AETT, with its convoluted use of fragrance to overcome undesirable or uncommercial odors, and a convenient decision to designate the ingredient as a fragrance, the public became its paying guinea pigs.

Included in the memorandum of the November 18, 1977, industry-FDA meeting was RIFM's agenda for its presentation to the agency. Last on the agenda was "Preparation of a position statement for the public." The public, however, received no statement until May 4, 1978, when the Environmental Defense Fund (EDF), a nonprofit, public-interest organization with 45,000 members, made public its letter to then FDA Commissioner Donald Kennedy asking for a ban on AETT use, ingredient disclosure by companies with products containing AETT, and FDA's informing the public of the hazard.

Industry's CTFA rushed a same-day statement lauding the industry's volunteerism.

The FDA issued no statement. Nor did it issue a statement when Leslie Dach, EDF's science associate, wrote another letter to Commissioner Kennedy on September 12, 1978, enclosing an abstract of Dr. Spencer's later findings in his continuing tests with AETT.

Dr. Spencer's tests with rats showed that AETT produced morphological effect "similar to those associated with a number of human neurological diseases, Canavan's disease, certain motor neuron diseases, vitamin B-12 deficiency, and toxic conditions produced by exposure to hexachlorophene and isoniazid."

The abstract described AETT as causing the splitting and bubbling of the nerve coverings of the spinal cord and brain, the disrupting of nerve impulses affecting motor coordination, progressive hyperirritability, and limb weakness. "Neuropathological changes accompanied the development of tissue discoloration and behavioral abnormalities." Damage to the nerve sheaths followed the development of excessive granules.

In a letter sent to EDF and quoted in Mr. Dach's letter to Commissioner Kennedy, Dr. Spencer concluded, "Please note that our new findings of neuronal ceroid degeneration add significantly to the public health hazard posed by this compound."

Commissioner Kennedy, however, answered Mr. Dach that "our information indicates that the problem is rapidly solving itself."

One wonders how many other unidentified "fragrance" ingredients are problems that are mysteriously "solving themselves" ... *how and on whom?* How many more unlisted, unidentified, and insufficiently tested "fragrance" ingredients are twenty-two-year-old problems "rapidly solving themselves"—ingredients that add nothing to the efficacy of products bought and used by consumers in the belief that they are safe.

QUESTIONS AND ANSWERS

Since I prefer to avoid fragrance ingredients, I bought the Wondra Skin Lotion labeled "UNSCENTED" instead of the one marked "REGULAR SCENT," thinking I was avoiding fragrance that might prove to be an allergen. When I got home and read the small print on the back label, I found that the "unscented" lotion had "masking *fragrance.*" Isn't this deceptive labeling?

I called Procter & Gamble, the company listed as Wondra's distributor, which means there probably is a manufacturer who remains unknown and undisclosed to the buyer-consumer. The reply to my question as to why an "unscented" product had an unexpected fragrance ingredient was: "Unscented products do have masking fragrance." (A check of other products labeled "unscented" showed that some did not include fragrance—masking or otherwise—in the ingredient list.)

When I pressed the fact that when an "unscented" product is bought, it is assumed that it is without fragrance, the explanation was that the masking fragrance was "to conceal the natural smell of the product, which would not be very good at all."

When I said that I didn't know that, and that I still expected no fragrance, the clever deflective labeling premise was explained.

Although the product was labeled "unscented," I was told: "It does have a fragrance that you can't detect. It's a masking fragrance, sort of like a neutralizing fragrance." (Actual sniffing, however, revealed that the product had a definite scent and was far from being neutral or without scent.)

When asked what the masking fragrance was, since my attempt to avoid fragrance was an attempt to avoid possible allergic reactions, I was told that the masking fragrance "had no special name to it" and asked what I was allergic to.

With this came the routine ploy used by most cosmetic companies you're likely to contact.

"If you can tell me what you're allergic to, I can contact our technical people and tell you if it's in there."

"I'd rather know what it is . . ."

"That's information we don't give out because it's formula information."

"But I'm allergic to fragrance . . ."

"What you need to do is to check with your doctor."

"In other words, you want me to tell you the answer for which I called you because the back label told me to call you if I had questions or comments."

After verbal dueling and circling back to the beginning, I pointed out that: (1) I was concerned that a supposedly unscented product contained fragrance ingredients, and (2) that AETT had a bad history as a masking fragrance, and I wanted to know if Wondra had, in the past, or has AETT in the unrevealed masking fragrance.

This piece of information was channeled to the "technical people," and I was called back and told that Wondra had not had and has no AETT.

With both the first and second department, I left the suggestion that Procter & Gamble try to come up with a lotion labeled "unscented" that was also *unfragranced* to comply with the perception of consumers who bought "unscented"-marked products because they preferred doing without fragrance ingredients.

Deceptive labeling? I'll leave that decision to the FDA. Language sleight of hand? Of course.

Wouldn't it be better if the cosmetic companies left the fragrance to the consumers to add in the form of perfumes and colognes if they wanted to smell that way, and let the consumers choose their fragrance and control its application, instead of putting questionable fragrance ingredients in a product that's going to be smeared all over the body?

Of course, but cosmetic companies are unconvinced that prospective buyers don't buy even a utilitarian product primarily on the fragrance.

The situation is similar to that of the food processors who salted everything in the theory that consumers demanded processed food to be heavily salted or it wouldn't taste good and there wouldn't be a repeat sale. Consumer education and subsequent demand blossomed into a spate of unsalted processed foods. Consumers were given a choice and allowed to use their own salt shaker according to their tastes.

The same progression was true of baby foods seasoned to please the mother, caffeined soft drinks, and canned fruit in thick, heavily sweetened syrup that suddenly emerged packed in its own juice, among other examples.

The formula for change is fairly simple: consumer education, followed by consumer demand for a choice, followed by industry realization of profits by supplying a choice. It's the old business of supply and demand—and it's up to you to make your demands known to the supplier.

I'm not a chemist, but "tetralin" brings up the rear of AETT (acetyl ethyl tetramethyl tetralin), and "Tetralin" is shown as a registered name for a chemical listed in *The Merck Index*. Its use is listed as a "degreasing agent and solvent for naphthalene, fats, resins, oils, waxes, used instead of turpentine in lacquers, shoepolishes, floorwaxes." The human toxicity is given as "May be irritating to skin, eyes and mucous membranes and, in high concentrations, narcotic. In experimental animals has produced cataracts and kidney injury." Could it be that anyone would add such an ingredient to a cosmetic?

It's a good question to ask those who might.

7

Color Additives–
The Battle of
the Quarter-Century

I would think that Congress might want to
consider establishing a definition of
negligible—say one estimated incremental cancer
death, lifetime, per million population.
—Donald Kennedy,
Former FDA Commissioner

A risk standard of one in one million is not
necessarily negligible. It would lead to an
additional 400 cancer deaths per year.
—Michael Jacobson,
Center for Science in the Public Interest

Rare in occurrence or not, it is not in any way
justified if it is preventable. Statistics are a poor
answer for the victim in whom the result has
been 100 percent hazardous.
—Dr. William J. Evans,
Formerly with FDA Bureau of Drugs

When the Delaney Hearings were convened to ex-
amine chemical additives in food, Congressman James J.
Delaney had no intention of including cosmetics in the hearings.
Hormones, however, were on the additives agenda,

since cattle were being treated with estrogenic hormones that were then turning up in beef—and the hormones had been found to cause cancer in animals.

One cosmetic formulator, who was using hormones in cosmetics, reportedly panicked at the thought that he might be forced to stop using estrogenic hormones in his cosmetic formulas. In an attempt to forestall the anticipated prohibition, the manufacturer called on Mr. Delaney.

According to another industry member, the congressman wasn't even aware of the existence of hormone cosmetics, and, at first, politely tried to brush off his caller. "Food was enough in the Delaney book. He wanted no part of cosmetics. But our friend insisted. He almost demanded that Mr. Delaney take additional testimony involving hormones in cosmetics."

And so the Delaney Committee opened the hearings to cosmetics and found out more than it cared to know. Consequently, the Delaney Hearings, with their belated inclusion of cosmetics, led to insecticide controls and the famous—or infamous, from industry's view—Delaney Amendment to the Food, Drug, and Cosmetic Act. The Delaney Amendment barred the use of any additive shown to cause cancer in man or beast. Cosmetics, however, were exempted and could continue to use estrogenic hormones that repeatedly had proved to cause cancer in animals.

A year before the hearings, however, children had become ill from eating Halloween popcorn candy colored with an unusually high concentration of FD&C Orange No. 1, an orange dye permitted for use in food, drugs, and cosmetics. In testing the color with newer pharmacological procedures, the FDA found that not only Orange No. 1 but many of the coal-tar dyes, formerly judged to be harmless, *were not harmless.*

Although samples from all batches of permitted coal-tar dyes are required to be checked for purity, certified, and numbered by the FDA before they are used in products, the original screening tests proved to have been inadequate.

Laboratory animals, fed formerly permitted dyes, developed ailments and injuries that included anemia, enlarged spleen, liver damage, and stunted growth. In some feeding tests death occurred in alarming percentages.

The first three colors found to be harmful were FD&C Orange Nos. 1 and 2 and Red No. 32. Hearing procedures to ban them took from 1953 to 1955, when children again became ill after eating popcorn "Halloween Cats" colored with FD&C Orange No. 1—the same dye that had caused illness five years before.

In November 1955, a final order removed the three colors from those permitted to be used in food. Unfortunately, it came too late to prevent nearly 200 people, most of them children, from becoming ill after eating popcorn colored with FD&C Red No. 32 during the Christmas season.

When fourteen other permitted coal-tar dyes did not pass the new tests, it became evident that further legislation was needed to protect consumers from eating dyes found no longer to be harmless. The dyes provided an ironic parallel in the bond between food and cosmetics. The same dyes were being used in foods for cosmetic reasons—to make strawberries appear redder, to dye eggless foods yellow to make them appear egg-filled—to fool the eye of the beholder so the beholder would become the buyer, much in the way Pavlov conditioned his dogs to react to a stimulus.

It took five years of legislative jousting through the hearing rooms and in the courts before the Color Additives Amendment was passed in 1960. Since the questionable dyes also were being used to color drugs *and* cosmetics—such as lipstick, which women ate along with their meals—the Color Additives Amendment included drugs and cosmetics.

The loudest protests came from the lipstick makers. They demanded to know what Congress was trying to do to the industry. Didn't Congress realize the industry couldn't carry on without those colors? There was bound to be a black market in illegal lipsticks, and all kinds of undesirables would emerge from the shadows!

The FDA, charged with administering the new amendment, insisted that, now, the cosmetic manufacturers had to test their colors and prove they were safe. They were being asked only to join the food and drug makers who had been doing some required testing and, despite this, had survived and flourished. Soaps and hair dyes, exempted from all regulation, continued exempt.

The significance of the 1960 Color Additives Amendment, however, went beyond being merely new regulation. For the first time, the burden of proof had slid onto the cosmetic industry's shoulders. Even though it was only for color additives, for the first time a cosmetic manufacturer would have to submit proof that an ingredient was *safe* before it was used in a cosmetic and marketed. No longer would it be fair game to chance the ingredient and the cosmetic until and unless the FDA caught up with it and proved it to be *unsafe*. It was also the first time cosmetics had been included in any addition to the Food, Drug, and Cosmetic Act since 1938.

After a few impassioned speeches given at industry meetings, describing the imminent revolt of American women deprived of their favorite lipstick shades (illustrated with films of London's wartime black market in cosmetics), the cosmetic industry settled down to the task of testing.

The 1960 Color Additives Amendment proved that premarket testing of ingredients need not be onerous. In fact, they proved that premarket testing was eminently workable when it is required and guidelines are established.

The FDA promptly made its test data on previous government-tested colors available to the industry. The cosmetic industry voluntarily dropped some questionable colors and eliminated others that weren't being used enough to warrant the expense of testing. The Pharmaceutical Manufacturers Association undertook the testing of several colors common to drugs and cosmetics. And the cosmetic industry, left with twenty-five colors to test, set up a cooperative testing program led by The Toilet Goods Association, now renamed The Cosmetic, Toiletry and Fragrance Association, otherwise referred to as CTFA.

The testing, involving two-year application and ingestion studies, was divided among five independent laboratories. The initial program extended over five years and reportedly cost the industry approximately one million dollars, paid by cosmetic companies on a use-assessment basis. Test data and reports were then evaluated by the FDA in establishing proof of the color's harmlessness for its intended use before being listed as approved.

The shared cost was modest when it is realized that almost a *billion dollars a year* was being spent just for television time and newspaper and magazine space to advertise cosmetic products. The long-overdue basic testing will serve the entire industry. Compared to the estimated $16.5 billion that was being collected annually from consumers for cosmetics and services, the cost of testing colors, which is reported to have risen to $7 million by 1979, hardly seems worth the lobbying fees the industry spent in fighting the amendment.

However, even though the forced testing of colors left over from those already approved for food and drugs provided a catalyst for the industry-CTFA coordinated effort to test other ingredients being used in cosmetics, almost a quarter of a century after the passage of the color amendment, the industry and the FDA are still dueling, delaying, and obstructing its implementation.

As CTFA explains it:

> In 1960, when Congress amended the federal Food, Drug, and Cosmetic Act to require pre-market safety clearance for colors, it established a system of "provisional" and "permanent" listing of color additives.
>
> During the 1960s and early 1970s, CTFA coordinated two rounds of tests to comply with color pre-market clearance requirements. However, the rapid advancement of technology prompted FDA to call for a third round of tests in 1977.
>
> By late 1982, CTFA had submitted to FDA reports on all but one of the 10 color additives for which the Association sponsored safety testing.

By 1983, the FDA had permanently listed twelve of the color additives culled from those submitted by CTFA. Eleven remained provisionally listed pending the outcome of the testing program. While the colors are provisionally listed, they may be continued to be used—as were many others during the nearly quarter of a century since the amendments were passed.

Although the cosmetic industry has enough dyes for Revlon to advertise a choice of 269 lipsticks and 127 nail polishes, and for one supplier to offer a choice of 111 eye shadows, CTFA promised its members to continue its efforts to maintain as wide a palette of cosmetic color additives as possible. While, for the innovative industry, this may seem laudable, an examination of the methods used to gain that objective brings to question whose safety is being protected.

According to CTFA:

> The Association plans not only to develop strategies to protect currently listed color additives but also to explore potential new uses for color additives now listed for limited use and consider the utility of color additives listed in Europe but not permitted for use in the United States. CTFA will also con-

sider re-petitioning FDA for color additives delisted in the past due to alleged contaminants.

The last sentence holds the clue to what has happened in Washington that has the cosmetic industry cheering the folks at the FDA. In effect, it opens the door to changing the Delaney clause from the theory that no amount of an ingredient that has been shown to cause cancer in man or beast is good for you to *maybe a little bit of a carcinogen might be okay if it's used to give the cosmetic industry one more dye to produce yet more shades of eyeshadow, lipstick or nail polish.*

The Delaney-clause breaker goes under the exotically phrased "trace constituents policy." CTFA calls it "FDA's Trace Constituents Policy"—as indeed it is.

The FDA announced its "trace constituents policy" in defense of its subsequent approval and permanent listing of color additives that did not live up to the "proved harmless" requirement of the 1960 Color Additives Amendment.

Against the stultifying inertia of the past two decades, the FDA, in comparatively rapid succession, permanently listed D&C Green No. 6, D&C Green, No. 5, and D&C Reds Nos. 6 & 7. All had p-toluidine, a known carcinogen, in their constituents.

The cosmetic industry, represented by the CTFA, applauded the move and "filed comments with FDA in support of the constituents policy."

According to Stephen H. McNamara, CTFA senior vice-president and general counsel, and formerly with the FDA: "The FDA has relied on its newly developed 'constituents policy.' Under this policy, FDA will not apply the Delaney anticancer clause to ban a color additive that contains an unwanted and unavoidable carcinogenic contaminant *if* the color itself (as distinguished from the unwanted 'constituent') is not carcinogenic, *and* use of the color (including the constituent) can be shown to present no significant human risk."

More simply—in the past—if an impurity that was an inherent part of the color additive was found to be a carcinogen, even though it was not part of the actual color, it could not be permanently listed as being safe for use.

The evidence for judging "no significant human risk," which the FDA decided was one more cancer victim per million people who, otherwise, might be spared cancer, was risk assessment studies provided by the industry.

The question remains: Given a choice, how many tax-paying consumers would opt for *any known risk* to maintain or enlarge a supplier's inventory of 111 different eye shadows—or to have a mouthwash in a particular shade of red?

And since the FDA plans to use the same "constituents policy" for food additives—would consumers, if asked, agree with the FDA that one life sacrificed to cancer in a million presents an acceptable "negligible risk" to color a fake-strawberry icing even though there are other reds available? Or to accommodate the industry with one more green to dye pistachio ice cream?

Dr. Michael Jacobson of the Center for Science in the Public Interest told a Senate Labor and Human Resources hearing that a risk standard of one in one million "is not necessarily negligible." The proposed FDA "acceptable" standard translated into an additional 400 cancer deaths a year.

The battle for the "constituents"—a word that used to refer to human beings represented by their legislators—brings to mind a comment made a number of years ago by Dr. William J. Evans, with the FDA Bureau of Drugs, in referring to eye injuries caused by contaminated eye products. His statement seems appropriate in the face of the FDA's new "constituents policy" and its companion "negligible risk assessment."

To quote Dr. Evans: "Rare in occurrence or not, it is not in any way justified if it is preventable. Statistics are a poor answer for the victim in whom the result has been 100 percent hazardous."

One consumer apparently agreed and felt strongly enough to take action. Glenn M. W. Scott, a Kentucky attorney, challenged the FDA's permanent listing of D&C Green No. 5 in the United States Court of Appeals for the Sixth Circuit Court in Cincinnati. "The Rose Sheet" of *FDC Reports,* a weekly trade newsletter, reported that Mr. Scott claimed that the FDA defended its action by arguing that p-toluidine, the carcinogenic constituent, is not a color additive and, therefore, not subject to the Delaney clause.

According to Mr. Scott: "FDA's point is irrelevant, we are dealing here not with p-toluidine by itself, but rather with D&C Green No. 5 . . . a mixture of several chemicals. Because the mixture contains a carcinogen, and use of the mixture will expose consumers to this carcinogen and the risk of cancer, the color additive cannot be legally listed."

Further, Mr. Scott claimed that FDA's approval of the dye on November 2, 1982, violated the Delaney clause. He pointed out that when the clause became part of the Color Additives law, the Secretary of Health, Education and Welfare explained that the clause was based on the simple fact that no one knows how to set a safe tolerance for substances in human foods when those substances are known to cause cancer when added to the diet of animals.

"This indicates clearly," the attorney concluded, "that Congress did not intend to put the FDA into the business of setting 'safe' tolerances for the carcinogen which is found in D&C Green No. 5. The FDA is now claiming the right to do that which Congress said could not be done."

The challenge went to court in June 1983 with an interesting sidelight. The CTFA, which usually appears against the

FDA, saw the litigation as a possible "test case" not only for D&C Green No. 5, but for determining the validity of the constituents policy as well. Consequently, it took the unusual step of notifying the court of its interest and was granted permission to appear in the litigation on an *amicus curiae* ("friend of the court") basis.

Meanwhile, back in Washington, the CTFA and FDA resumed their dueling. This time the dueling involved carcinogens that the FDA claimed were in the actual colors and not just in the constituents, on which the agency had already yielded. If carcinogens were found to be in the actual color, the color additive would be expressly forbidden by the Delaney clause to the 1960 Color Additives Amendment.

As E. Edward Kavanaugh, CTFA president, expressed it, the FDA "in effect, is not willing to make any scientific judgment about these color additives. What they're saying is that 'we want more tests, we want more tests, we want more tests.' We're going to have to spend more money and waste more money; and then they're going to say at the end, 'If there's any risk at all, even if there's one in 50 *billion*,' which is what we're showing, 'then we're going to remove the color from the market under the Delaney clause.' "

Reminded that the FDA had already approved colors with carcinogens found in the constituents, Mr. Kavanaugh said, "Yes, when there is a constituent. Now [in] some of these cases, they're arguing that it's the color itself that may be having a carcinogenic effect in the rats or the mice. And what we're saying is—it doesn't make any difference because the risk is infinitesimal and we've spent thousands and thousands of dollars with some of the Harvard researchers and others projecting a risk assessment. In other words, what is the risk to a human. And it's crazy. You're talking about one-in-16-billion lifetime risk and FDA is saying, 'Well, if it's one in a hundred billion, it doesn't make any difference; because if it's one in anything, the Delaney clause says we have to remove it from the market.' And that is just a lot of poppycock. It's ridiculous."

As a consumer, I told Mr. Kavanaugh that I was on the other side; and speaking for the consumer, "We are bombarded on all sides. We take risks in all cases. However, with 150 colors just in eye shadows, and they say they have God knows how many lipstick shades—for one more shade, is it worth it to have even the battle, *even the money* that's being spent on this?

"Then the color additive goes into food where it's all clumped together [as unidentified 'certified color']. Okay, the risk is minimal; I accept that. But I keep hearing about lotteries where your chances are one in five, six, sixteen million. And yet there's a winner. Somebody always wins that prize."

"Right," Mr. Kavanaugh conceded, "but in this case, this risk assessment does not mean that it's ever going to happen."

"We don't know that," I said. "From a consumer's standpoint—if it's a necessary risk, okay—our life is a risk. However, if it's a risk to make one other shade that is so infinitesimally different when you have all of these shades already, and just to make, say, a strawberry look redder or to make something that doesn't have eggs look as though it has eggs in it . . ."

Mr. Kavanaugh explained that, obviously, one color would generate many shades; and ten years ago, the industry had 80 or 84 colors available. In 1983, the number was down to 36.

"And they still can get 150 shades of eye shadow."

"Yes, but if we start losing these basic red colors . . . then it's going to drastically affect how the industry can formulate their products."

"And if you go back to find a shade you like, you can't find it, because they're pushing something new."

"That's often true. I agree with that."

I reminded Mr. Kavanaugh that the industry should have been testing its ingredients long before the 1960 Color Additives Amendment forced it into its color-testing program. Then, too, the program was reasonable, and none of the companies seemed to be going bankrupt because of it.

"Also," I added, "I think the cosmetic industry is innovative enough and bright enough to come out with whatever it needs with whatever it is that it has. It will think of a way of doing it."

I pointed out that perhaps the men who control the industry, government, and agencies were so busy talking to each other that they were not as aware as they should be of the growing concern among consumers, and that most women could easily do without 160 shades of eye shadow instead of 150 and without 300 shades of lipstick.

I also took the opportunity to suggest to the CTFA president that a lot of problems could be solved and a tremendous amount of time and expense saved by all, including the underwriting taxpaying consumers, if the cosmetic industry would make do with the colors already approved and go on with its business. After all, a quarter of a century of jousting should be enough for anyone.

QUESTIONS AND ANSWERS

Why is it that we consumers seem to get so little news about activities going on that will directly effect our lives while so much is made of politicians making public appearances and speeches?

Visibility makes the difference. A politician cutting a ribbon to open a bridge or making a speech to prospective voters is more visible and easier to cover than unannounced meetings, court hearings, and tacit agreements.

Also, most reporters are generalists, as are most congressmen; and it takes a special knowledge of the subject to ask the questions that will elicit the information that is required.

How can a consumer become aware of coming changes or proposed actions before they're an accomplished fact?

Often with difficulty. For instance, FDA statements of intent are published in the *Federal Register*. Few consumers do or should subscribe to the *Federal Register*. It's expensive, bulky, and boring. And you'd have to wade through a lot of political speeches, some not even spoken, but handed in to impress what used to be called the "constituents" back home.

Otherwise, you'd need access to industry trade publications and insider newsletters, which are not as boring as the *Federal Register,* but much more expensive and harder to get.

The best way to keep informed is to join a consumer organization that monitors the various branches of government and regularly reports to its members. We must realize that what we find on our store shelves is the result of what goes on in Washington as well as in the conduit that fills the shelves.

How can we make our views known before a proposal becomes law?

Once an agency, such as the FDA, publishes its proposed action or regulation, a period of time is given for comment. Comments can be made by anyone, and they are evaluated. In the case of the Kentucky lawyer, Glenn Scott, he persisted into the courts. Sometimes you win, sometimes you lose, but at least you have an opportunity to prove you're a *human* constituent who cares about not wanting to swallow the FDA carcinogenic constituent the agency wants to force-feed an entire nation.

Additional tip: Legislators are more vulnerable than regulators—and, usually, they're particularly willing to listen during election years. The more constituents who reach them the better. If they're the right ones for your vote, they'll *want* to be informed. Organizations and numbers count. The more visibility you can get, the better. If you can tell your tale well, even the media will listen.

8

Deregulation-Not Just Another Pretty Word

Of all FDA activities, the only FDA activity that enjoys a lower priority than cosmetics is the Board of Tea Tasters, under the Tea Importation Act.
—**Professor Joseph A. Page,**
Georgetown University Law Center

Donald A. Davis, editor of *Drug & Cosmetic Industry,* a leading trade magazine, has been a cosmetics watcher for more than twenty years. When asked what he thought was of highest import in the field of cosmetics in the 1980s, he answered with one word: "Deregulation."

"I think the most important thing that has happened since the beginning of the eighties is deregulation, for obvious reasons. It has pulled the teeth of the FDA as an effective agency.

"Even when they do recalls, now they're very, very careful not to offend or hurt anybody. Some of their relations with the industry have gotten much easier for both. They have, in effect, pretty much ignored the consumer movement—at least, since about the latter part of 1982."

When asked why he chose that time, he said, "Well, it took about a year for the deregulation to take effect. For instance, the old FDA commissioner was there about five or six months after Reagan got into office."

Reminded of the time George P. Larrick was the FDA commissioner for what seemed to be a lifetime in the 1960s, before commissioners were quickly going through a revolving door, Don Davis replied, "Those days are gone. It's become a very political office now."

Getting back to deregulation, he said, "That's the most important thing—the thing that's bothered me the most as a journalist—because, in effect, a lot of what the FDA does has been short-circuited."

In September 1981, Heinz J. Eiermann, director of FDA's Division of Cosmetics Technology, had already acknowledged that "regulation by federal agencies has been undergoing a major change in direction. The seeds of this change were planted years ago; they have come into bloom during the past twelve months."

"Overregulation," he noted, "has been a favorite subject of public discussion for many years. The current [Reagan] administration has made regulatory reform, including deregulation, a high-priority goal. On February 17, 1981, in Executive Order 12291, the President ordered federal agencies not to undertake regulatory action 'unless the potential benefits to society for the regulation outweigh the potential costs to society.' The President also ordered agencies to base administration decisions on 'adequate information concerning the need for and consequences of proposed government action' and to choose 'among alternative approaches to any given regulatory objective, the alteration involving the least net cost to society.'

"To implement the President's order, an agency is required to prepare a regulatory impact analysis in connection with every existing or proposed major rule. The purpose of the analysis is to determine whether a new rule meets the criteria of the Executive Order and, applying the same criteria, whether a currently effective rule should be retained without change, modified, or revoked."

"It is apparent," Mr. Eiermann added, "that rulemaking has become a rather intricate and burdensome process in the United States. Moreover, the requirement for periodic review of existing regulations will place additional, sizable demands on the already scarce resources of the cosmetics program."

After listing the several steps the FDA had attempted to take in an effort to protect consumers from cosmetic ingredients that had been proven harmful, and then being forced to scrap proposed label warnings or the banning of unsafe ingredients, Mr. Eiermann concluded: "We have entered a new era in regulatory activity in the United States which places a major new burden on regulatory agencies. Although consumer protection remains the determining factor for taking action against hazardous products or activities, rulemaking no longer is the obvious choice for solving safety problems. The new requirements placed upon regulatory agencies demand exhaustive analysis of avenues other than rulemaking, and the proposal of a regulation has become the last resort to achieve the intended effect."

Mr. Eiermann's comments might have been of interest to American consumers, many of whom have yet to realize how deregulation is directly affecting them and how it will increasingly affect the quality of American life. Unfortunately, his comments were made in Copenhagen, Denmark, at the conference of the International Federation of Societies of Cosmetic Chemists.

In mid-April 1983, the heads of the U.S. Executive Departments and Agencies received a lengthy bulletin from the

Executive Office of the President, Office of Management and Budget (OMB), signed by its director, David A. Stockman. Subject: *Fiscal Year 1984 Information Collection Budget Request.*

The mild-sounding heading masked incendiary directives in language more appropriate to army commands. Under the guise of "paperwork reduction," begun with the "Paperwork Reduction Act of 1980," Mr. Stockman announced that some changes had been made.

The bulletin warned:

> Agencies should note that the definition of "collection of information" has been revised substantially to include items such as procurement, disclosure, labeling, and testing requirements.

The following month, *Food Chemical News* reported that former Secretary of Health and Human Services Richard S. Schweiker "had stongly opposed the Office of Management and Budget's proposal for OMB clearance of labeling requirements under the Paperwork Reduction Act." Secretary Schweiker, who headed the overall agency of the FDA, had submitted comments to the OMB on its proposed implementation of the Act and Executive Order, but his comments apparently were ignored in shaping the final regulations.

Secretary Schweiker claimed the Office of Management and Budget had expanded the definition of the term "collection of information" to include vital requirements such as labeling that went beyond the intention of Congress when it passed the Paperwork Reduction Act. The secretary contended that the OMB's insistence that agencies routinely obtain clearances for such requirements would result in a substantial increase in internal agency paperwork and delays in the conduct of department business.

According to Secretary Schweiker, "The Act does not cover requirements to disclose information to the public and, thus, the proposed rule could be justified only if labeling were viewed as a recordkeeping requirement."

The Secretary was not alone in questioning the OMB's legal authority for many of its proposals. Other agencies, among them the Justice Department, also claimed that OMB had exceeded its intended authority.

For cosmetic regulation, already the impoverished relative of the FDA, deregulation was an all-but-fatal blow.

Trade editor Don Davis said, "There's even talk that the truth-in-labeling business will be either suppressed or discontinued."

Referring to David Stockman's signing of the April 1983 bulletin, he added, "He is trying to alleviate what industry has to put out ... to use a strange expression ... in terms of co-operating with its regulatory agencies."

While the cosmetic industry and its many Washington representatives go on creating more and more paperwork as they prepare endless layers of challenges, court briefs, and risk-assessment studies in what appears to be an attempt to create an oasis of laissez-faire, David Stockman's decree already seems to have cowed the tiny office of cosmetic regulators.

Ironically, while Mr. Stockman was busy dismembering consumer-protective regulations so that little, if any, recordkeeping or "paperwork" would be required from industry, the cosmetic industry, for one, was creating mountains of unrequired paperwork and forcing the former regulators more and more to become recordkeepers.

And while the cosmetics regulatory branch has been reduced to a mere twig, the industry's most prominent representative, The Cosmetic, Toiletry and Fragrance Association, has rivaled Jack's proverbial beanstalk by sprouting from a two-man office in New York City, which is surrounded by most of the cosmetic companies, to almost sixty employees based in Washington, D.C., which is devoid of known cosmetic companies.

A nonprofit organization, CTFA did not include a financial statement in its annual report; but it is safe to assume that its annual budget would swallow the $2.47 million allocated for the 1983 FDA budget for the entire cosmetic program.

In the face of severe inflation, while other programs were being increased, the cosmetics program was cut from $2.979 million in 1978, to $2.044 million in 1979, to $1.855 million in 1980.

Less than seven tenths of one percent of FDA's 1983 total annual budget of $356 million was allocated to monitoring an industry that is surpassed only by the food industry in the number of products sold yearly and used daily by the entire population throughout entire lifetimes.

The $2.47 million budget provided salaries for a total of fifty-six man years, including seventeen man years in the Washington headquarters and eight man years in the field for cosmetic inspections. The $2.47 million also had to cover everything else spent on the program, including travel expenses for court appearances and speechmaking, as well as the day-to-day expenditures of monitoring and trying to regulate an industry whose sales in 1982 exceeded $12.5 *billion.*

Meanwhile, over on Vermont Avenue in the District of Columbia, the CTFA solicited enough funds from its members, through its Political Action Committee, to support the campaigns of eleven candidates running for seats in the House of Representatives in the 1982 fall election. The CTFA told its members in its annual report: "All made successful bids to return to office."

The Fall 1982 issue of *CTFA Cosmetic Journal,* CTFA's quarterly magazine, depicted another contest. This time, the contest was an illustrated game of tennis. A regulation-sized tennis ball was shown going *through* a teal-blue net. The ball grew larger as it curved downward, even larger as it spiraled up to the facing page and on to fill almost half a page as it landed in industry's court.

The article illustrated was titled: "The Ball's In Industry's Court." The author, shown smiling in a photograph, was John A. Wenninger, deputy director, Division of Cosmetics Technology, Food and Drug Administration.

Referring to one of the unsolved problems with nitrosamine contamination in cosmetics, which presented yet another carcinogenic risk to consumers, Mr. Wenninger concluded: "We will continue our cooperative efforts with the CTFA in this area. However, it is very doubtful that we can maintain the level of scientific resources that we have devoted to this area in the past. Most of the research in this area may have to be done by industry, not government."

And that was written *before* David Stockman sent his bulletin around.

QUESTIONS AND ANSWERS

How do I go about finding a consumer organization that represents my interests?

The news is your best source. Make a note of the organizations that testify in congressional hearings, the representatives of organizations called upon to comment on the issues that interest you, and those hardy souls who speak and act according to beliefs that match your own.

What if I can't find an organization that shares my concern?

Start your own. Many large and successful organizations began with one person. Check around and you'll find you're not alone in your concern. Someone is waiting for the other person to take the initiative. You're the other person.

How much good does writing to senators and congressmen do?

A great deal—especially when the mail and/or telegrams pile up from registered or prospective voters. A postmark from one of their districts is a magic emblem.

If I happen to be in Washington, can I drop in and see my senator or representative?

It helps to make an appointment. If your legislator can't see you at that time, arrangements usually can be made for you to see a staff member. However, I have seen a senator, who had just completed hearings based on my investigations, and who I was told would be "tied up" indefinitely, shoot out of his office to greet an unknown constituent who had apologetically mentioned to the receptionist that he was just passing through Washington and it wasn't necessary to disturb the senator if he was busy. But then, it *was* an election year, and I was from another state.

9

The "Self-Regulated" Industry

The Ball's in Industry's Court.
—John A. Wenninger,
Deputy Director,
Division of Cosmetics Technology,
Food and Drug Administration

In 1979, the Cosmetic Ingredient Review, a program begun by the Cosmetic, Toiletry and Fragrance Association at the time ingredient labeling became law, won an award. A Consumer Product Safety Award was given to it by the National Association of Professional Insurance Agents.

The Cosmetic Ingredient Review (CIR) defines itself as "a voluntarily formed scientific safety evaluation organization. Its single purpose is to make determinations concerning the safety of cosmetic ingredients." Its procedures "include evaluation of available published and unpublished information on an ingredient by a panel of expert scientists and clinicians, and the issuance of a report that is offered for public comment before being finalized."

The CIR was planned as an independent entity. Its

panel members must neither be employed nor funded by the cosmetic industry. However, its steering committee consists mostly of CTFA executives, and it is totally dependent on the CTFA for its support.

In 1982, the CIR annual budget of $500,000 was augmented by $150,000 to fund clinical studies needed when there was insufficient data. Nevertheless, the CIR is primarily a data collection agency, rather than a testing arm of the industry, as is the CTFA-sponsored color additives program. According to the CIR Sourcebook, the decision on an ingredient's safety can be put aside when insufficient data is found.

In addition to the steering committee and an independent expert panel, three nonvoting members are selected, one each from industry, a consumer organization, and the FDA.

According to the lengthy and involved procedures, the nonvoting liaison representatives "shall not have access to confidential data and information that are not available for public disclosure ... shall not be present at any portion of an Expert Panel meeting that is closed for the presentation of confidential data ... shall not make any presentation to the Expert Panel during a hearing conducted by the Expert Panel ... shall exercise restraint in performing his functions and shall not engage in unseemly advocacy or attempt to exert undue influence over members of the Expert Panel."

Given all the shall-nots, it is debatable that the consumer representative can be anything more than window dressing. On the other hand, the industry representative has access to pertinent information, if needed, as does the FDA contact person who can call on the agency's resources.

The CTFA is to be congratulated for its concept of having a peer group study the available data on various ingredients used by its members in their products. Given its limitations, the CIR provides a helpful tool for the industry in avoiding duplication of gathering and reviewing literature on selected ingredients.

As CTFA explains: "While CIR cannot diminish the need for manufacturers to evaluate the safety of finished products, it can reduce the amount of independent testing necessary for individual ingredients and provide data otherwise unavailable to industry."

In other words, there is a great deal more to making a cosmetic safe. There is the matter of percentages used, combinations of chemicals, the methods of production, sanitation, contamination, stability ... and it is the finished product that reaches the consumer.

There are other limitations inherent in CTFA's Cosmetic Ingredient Review. Only a fraction of the approximately 3,000 CTFA-listed cosmetic ingredients are evaluated by CIR. Another estimate of ingredients used by the cosmetic industry is about 8,000 in more than 25,000 formulations under more than 50,000 brand names. Considering that just one private-label supplier advertised that it had "over 5,000 products and packages from 60 suppliers," one realizes the extent of cosmetics proliferation.

CIR's "initial priority list" selected 189 ingredients for review. According to the CIR 1982 Annual Report, 6 final reports on 13 cosmetic ingredients were issued by the expert panel during 1982, bringing the total to 36 final reports on 92 ingredients since the inception of the program in 1976. In addition, there were 12 tentative reports on 57 ingredients.

The Fall 1982 issue of CTFA Cosmetic Journal gave a different total of 43 final or tentative reports on 133 ingredients and claimed the ingredients were "all considered safe," leaving the reader to wonder why some reports remained "tentative."

The CTFA Cosmetic Journal article, "The CIR Story:

Big Cog in Cosmetic Industry Self-Regulatory Machine" states, "While Panel approval does not guarantee the safety of an ingredient, approval does confer reasonable assurance that the ingredient is safe under current conditions."

Yet, in another paragraph, CTFA's Director Gerald McEwen, Jr., is quoted as saying that self-regulation demonstrates to consumers that industry is interested in offering only safe products and "is willing to develop programs to ensure that safety without being forced to do so by government."

But in *CIR & Industry: A Sourcebook,* the admission is made: "It is also true that CTFA's creation of CIR occurred in response to growing consumer activist, congressional and regulatory agency pressure to increase regulation of cosmetic products."

The program, in fact, was not begun until ingredient labeling became mandatory. The effect of law versus voluntary "self-regulation" is evident in the fact that color additives, which must be proved safe before they are used in cosmetics, are being tested by the CTFA on behalf of the industry. Other ingredients, for which no premarket testing, is legally required, are being given literature reviews for a token number. Even when the expert panel trickles down its decision of safety, the safety is not guaranteed.

Since the expert panel is largely dependent on published material and whatever those in industry choose to channel to it, there is the nagging question of whether a company that has discovered something amiss with an ingredient would share its finding if it has a million or so units containing that ingredient in the market.

It is not unusual for a company to report a problem years after receiving consumer complaints and realizing it had a problem, apparently only when it becomes convenient to announce that it is discontinuing the offender. Information can then be funneled to the proper government officials. It will be relatively easier, at that time, to agree that all products—especially competing products—should be recalled and the ingredient banned.

Despite delays, if a federal agency, such as the FDA, considers the matter to be a serious threat to consumers, it *has* the power to seize the products, to order a recall, to ban the use of an ingredient, to issue warnings, or to take whatever action may be appropriate.

The CTFA or the CIR can do none of this. The most it can do is to make recommendations to members, send out publicity releases, and have meetings with government officials to try to persuade them to do nothing.

Of course, it helps to know as much as possible about what the manufacturers are putting into their products. The shame is that so little was known and so little was done to try to know that it took the force of legislation for the ingredients to be disclosed at all.

Now that cosmetic ingredients must be listed, the specter of one day having to explain them has prompted self-protective actions that are sailing under the guise of "self-regulation."

CIR brandishes the amorphous threat of substantiating safety or otherwise confessing on each label that the safety of the ingredients or the product has not been determined. According to its sourcebook, "CIR provides information for substantiating the safety of ingredients, and the conclusions of a panel of recognized, independent experts to meet this requirement." Again, it glides over the "finished product" substantiation.

About "affecting" legislation: "Although CIR actions have not directly affected federal legislation to date, CIR is, in part, a response to proposed congressional action to expand regulation of cosmetics. Much of the proposed legislation included requirements for specific premarket testing and clearance by FDA.

"However, since the inception of CIR, no legislation relating to safety testing of cosmetic ingredients has been introduced ..."

Allowing that the CTFA speaks the loudest for the cosmetic industry, the CTFA described its membership as including more than 250 companies that manufacture or distribute finished cosmetic products marketed in the United States and 230 associate member companies from related industries, such as manufacturers of cosmetic raw materials and packaging materials.

The FDA estimates that there are at least 2,000 known cosmetic companies. Since registration with the FDA is not required, guesses range upward to double the FDA estimate.

So, while the CTFA and CIR serve CTFA's members well in compiling basic information on ingredients that have been in use and in the market, they neither speak for nor reach the many cosmetic companies going their own way with their own rules or nonrules. Many of these companies may never have heard of CIR or ingredient and product substantiation or warning labels or ...

More accurately, the industry, led by the CTFA, is practicing self-protection rather than self-regulation. As a steering committee for *part* of the industry, which it claims accounts for 90 percent of the cosmetics sold in the country, CTFA has accomplished the extraordinary feat of bringing the cosmetic industry into the twentieth century.

With the advent of ingredient labeling, the CTFA compiled thousands of ingredients used in cosmetics, standardized the nomenclature, and published the first edition of the *CTFA Cosmetic Ingredient Dictionary* in 1973. Conceived by Norman Estrin, CTFA's senior vice-president in charge of science, the impressive work was planned in coordination with James M. Akerson, then with Gillette Medical Evaluation Laboratories.

To fully appreciate what must have been a herculean task, one must realize that, prior to ingredient labeling, cosmetic ingredients did not have to be disclosed, so it mattered little what the ingredients were called by the myriad companies and suppliers. The dictionary lists the chemical names and trade names of each ingredient, along with the CTFA-adopted name and a definition of the ingredient.

Recognition of the *CTFA Cosmetic Ingredient Dictionary* by the FDA as the source of ingredient nomenclature for product labeling made it the definitive industry reference and paved the way for updating and expanding subsequent editions. The third edition, published in 1982, is an oversized hardcover book of 610 tightly printed pages, includes 20,000 chemical and trade names, and is dedicated to "the world's consumers, as a continuing expression of The Cosmetic Industry's appreciation of consumer needs and desires."

In addition to the industry's definitive ingredient dictionary, the CTFA has published a step-by-step labeling manual and a number of other reference works. It also has begun, on a reasonable and collective basis, to do *some* testing for the industry and to provide *some* information that the industry should have had all along.

As admirable as CTFA's efforts to educate and modernize may be, they are closer to *self-education* than to "self-regulation"—just as the creation of the Cosmetic Ingredient Review is, more plainly, *self-protection* for the cosmetic industry in preparation for the day when the public may possibly become informed and begin to ask rude questions. Without appropriate answers, consumers may again become "activists" and the *entire* industry may again be faced with "growing consumer activist, congressional and regulatory agency pressure to increase regulation of cosmetic products" that started the "CTFA's creation of CIR" in the first place.

It is significant that the Consumer Product Safety Award was given to CTFA's Cosmetic Ingredient Review by the National Association of Professional Insurance Agents. Any step to cut down on those pesky and expensive out-of-court settlements brought on by injured and provoked consumers is a step to be applauded and encouraged . . . particularly by insurance agents. For consumers, it is just that—*a step.* Important, yes; "self-regulation," no.

As one wag was heard to say, "A laxative is the only self-regulation that's been known to work."

QUESTIONS AND ANSWERS

Does the Cosmetic Ingredient Review Expert Panel also decide which cosmetic ingredients are harmful and should be discontinued?

A search of the provisions in *CIR & Industry: A Sourcebook* found only provisions for determining safety. However, the 1982 CTFA Annual Report states, "Each report must reach one of three conclusions—there is a reasonable certainty that the ingredient is safe under conditions of use, it is unsafe, or there is insufficient data to make a judgment."

Has the CIR found any of the selected ingredients to be unsafe?

According to the CTFA: "To date [1983], the panel has found no ingredient unsafe, although it has proposed reasonable limits on the use of certain ingredients."

Does the CIR test the ingredients?

No. However, beginning in 1982, the CTFA has allocated $150,000 to be used for testing ingredients when the expert panel finds that the collected data is insufficient for determining the ingredient's safety. When testing is necessary, the CTFA usually arranges to have an outside laboratory do the testing.

‾ 10 ‾
Voluntary–The Magic Word

Vol-un-tar-y: proceeding from or regulated
by the will.
—**Webster's Dictionary**

Originally, cosmetic ingredient labeling was voluntary. It didn't work. Then a funny thing happened on the way to regulation.

Professor Joseph A. Page, then an associate professor at Georgetown University Law Center in Washington, D.C., was looking for a new, unexplored, and neglected subject for his Lawyering in the Public Interest Seminar.

The Page search for a subject coincided with the publication of my first book, *Cosmetics: Trick or Treat?* In it, I questioned, among other things, the ratio of risk to benefit of questionable cosmetics—some with known carcinogens, acknowledged sensitizers, irritants, contaminants, suspected nerve and brain toxins, ingredients with the possibility of causing systemic damage and birth defects—none of which were required to be tested or cleared before being loosed in million- and billion-unit promotions on the uninformed general public.

As a cosmetic consumer, I asked why ingredients of products used intimately by the entire population, from infancy and throughout daily life, should not be revealed and listed on labels as were the ingredients of other staples, from dog food to mattresses.

By late 1960 and early 1970, my book had gone into a number of editions and had attracted the attention of Joe Page, a Harvard classmate and friend of Ralph Nader. In it, he found the subject for his graduate-student seminar.

The Page Seminar was begun with Anthony L. Young, who met with me and impressed me with his comprehensive understanding of the subject, and several other students in August 1971. The seminar concentrated on using the combined legal and investigative skills to become the cosmetics watchdog for consumers in Washington.

According to Professor Page, "A look at the legislative and administrative framework of cosmetic regulation as it existed when the Seminar commenced its activity revealed a law with serious weaknesses and loopholes, and regulatory area that was given low priority status at the FDA."

Previously, in 1966, the same year in which the first edition of *Cosmetics: Trick or Treat?* appeared, Congress had passed the Fair Packaging and Labeling Act.

During the Senate hearings on the bill in 1963, George P. Larrick, then FDA commissioner, testified, "The cosmetic chapter of the Food, Drug, and Cosmetic Act does not require label information about the ingredients of cosmetics.

"Under the bill the Government would be empowered to require information about cosmetic ingredients where this is necessary to establish or preserve fair competition by enabling consumers to make rational comparisons with respect to price and other qualities or to prevent the deception of consumers.

"We believe it is as important that cosmetic labeling contain statements of ingredients as it is that many of the consumer commodities controlled by the Federal Trade Commission's regulations give this information. For example, some cosmetics contain ingredients that sensitize. This would justify a declaration of their presence on the label so that consumers who are sensitive to them may purchase other products less likely to cause rash or other reaction."

But, in 1966, when the bill became law, cosmetic ingredients remained undisclosed and unlabeled. There was a new commissioner at the FDA, and as the late Stephen L. Mayham, who was the voice of the industry for twenty-five years, said, "They pass a law and then they forget all about it."

If the agency had forgotten the Fair Packaging and Labeling Act it had wanted so it could give consumers the right to choose their cosmetics by reading the ingredients on the labels, the industry had not. The industry saw it as a Damocles sword and scurried to prevent its descent.

The Cosmetic, Toiletry and Fragrance Association, formerly the Toilet Goods Association, also had a new head man. With increased staff and dues, the TGA-CTFA moved from New York City and the heart of the cosmetic industry to Washington, D.C., where the commuting time to the agencies was minutes instead of hours. The little industry, which had begun with a few enterprising women cooking up a mess of goo in bathtubs and garages, had arrived in Washington as big business with lots of dollars from high-profit companies to buy the best and the brightest.

Among the brightest was Peter Barton Hutt of the prestigious law firm of Covington and Burling, known for representing leading food, drug, and cosmetic interests in their dueling with government agencies. Peter Barton Hutt became the CTFA counsel and is credited with engineering the "voluntary" system that was to masquerade as "self-regulation." It was a brilliant concept, and its orchestration charmed the FDA not only into agreeing to forego implementing the Fair Packaging and Labeling Act with cosmetic ingredient labeling, but also into publishing CTFA's voluntary labeling proposal as its FDA "regulation."

CTFA's beguiling offer of volunteering went beyond labeling. On August 26, 1971, the FDA published the package of "voluntary regulations" for the cosmetic industry proposed by the CTFA. Five days later, CTFA's counsel, Peter Hutt, moved to the FDA as FDA's general counsel.

In a farcical game of musical chairs, William W. Goodrich, who until June 1971 had been FDA's chief legal counsel, retired suddenly after thirty-three years of government service. At the same time, he suggested that a former student of a food and drug law course he taught be hired as his replacement.

Billy Goodrich's former student was Peter Barton Hutt, who, as a member of Covington and Burling, had been CTFA's legal counsel for the past two years and, reportedly, was the architect of the "voluntary," nonregulatory plan. Previously, Mr. Hutt had been the legal counsel for the Institute of Shortening and Edible Oils, a food trade association.

At about the same time, Mr. Goodrich was appointed president of the Institute of Shortening and Edible Oils, a former adversary as well as the former employer of his former pupil and present choice for his FDA replacement.

As Mr. Hutt slid into Mr. Goodrich's chair and Mr. Goodrich left for Mr. Hutt's former workplace, New York Congressman Benjamin S. Rosenthal, since deceased, remarked, "It looks like a game of musical chairs."

Mr. Hutt's volunteering to disqualify himself from actions in which he or his former law firm had been "substantially involved" led Congressman Rosenthal to add: "He has represented every food and drug client imaginable. He is going to have to disqualify himself from 75 percent of the cases coming before the FDA in the next few years."

James S. Turner, a Naderite who wrote *The Chemical Feast,* was reported as saying that it was unfair to subject Hutt to a private struggle with his conscience over "substantial" regulatory issues, particularly since "when his conscience loses, the public will never know."

Despite the protests; despite the public hearing called by Senator Frank E. Moss of Utah, who said, "We cannot continue to take people from the regulated and make them the regulators"; and despite the many who found it hard to believe that, of all the brilliant, dedicated lawyers in the nation, the FDA could only find one who, according to Washington nutritionist Robert Choate, came "from the very group of lawyers most adept at tying up the FDA's regulatory processes"—Peter Barton Hutt reported on schedule to the office vacated by his old instructor, adversary, and endorser, William W. Goodrich.

In excusing himself from participating in further shepherding the proposed "voluntary regulations," Mr. Hutt left the taxpaying consumers without the services of its chief FDA counsel, who presumably had been appointed to protect consumers from the very games played by the fox who was now in the chicken coop along with all of us chickens.

By May 1975, a scant four years after he became chief counsel for the FDA, and with the voluntary nonregulations still firmly in place, Mr. Hutt resigned. He quickly returned to Covington and Burling, a more valuable partner with firsthand, inside knowledge of the very agency whose regulatory processes Covington and Burling "was most adept at tying up."

In the seduction of the FDA by the CTFA, the resulting

voluntary "regulations" paradoxically protected the industry while stripping consumers of the right to know what they were using on or in their bodies in their normal routine of cleansing, grooming, and one would hope beautifying.

According to the volunteered "regulations," cosmetic companies could *volunteer* to register with the FDA so they could be found by FDA inspectors who already knew where many of them were. Since there was no requirement to register, even members of the CTFA were free *not to volunteer.*

Cosmetic companies could also *volunteer* to tell the FDA what they had put into their products, but the industry-proposed "regulations" allowed every company to remain free *not to volunteer.* Even then, the volunteers were excused from revealing the flavors and fragrances, or any "trade secret" ingredients they used in their products. Those who were magnanimous enough to list their "trade secrets" with the FDA would be rewarded with an ironclad pledge that not only the FDA, but also physicians seeking information to help patients discover the cause of their allergies and injuries, would keep the identity of the ingredients secret.

In effect, the CTFA-FDA had made it possible for the cosmetic industry to continue with its unique mandate to keep consumers ignorant of the ingredients in family staples such as toothpaste and shampoo, as well as $25-an-ounce face creams and the latest shade of nail polish.

Fortunately for consumers, the Page Seminar in Lawyering in the Public Interest was in session. A petition, signed by Professor Page and Anthony L. Young, was filed to make cosmetic ingredient labeling mandatory under the Fair Packaging and Labeling Act. The Consumer Federation of America joined as a copetitioner of what was to become the basis for the cosmetic ingredient labeling regulation. The transition from petition to the effective labeling date took about five years.

Although the loopholes remain in the nondisclosure of fragrances and flavors, trade secrets, and the ingredients in cosmetic products not intended to be sold directly to consumers, the Page-Young victory provided the FDA with, at least, some rudimentary tools.

Left as voluntary were the registration of manufacturing and packing establishments, reporting of cosmetic raw materials and cosmetic ingredients in finished product formulations, and cosmetic product experiences including information about adverse reactions.

As of 1980, 950 cosmetic companies had registered with the FDA, out of more than 2,000 known companies and thousands more throughout the country not yet discovered by the FDA in Washington. Approximately 3,600 raw materials and 19,500 finished-product formulations were reported out of about 8,000 known chemical entities, and at least 25,000 known formulations and more than 50,000 brand names. When it comes to filing information about adverse reactions—the most important to injured or about-to-be-injured consumers—only about 70 companies have volunteered.

In 1983, despite the FDA's streamlining the voluntary report forms so that a minimum of information could be given, Commissioner Arthur Hull Hayes, Jr., told industry members gathered in Boca Raton for their annual convention, "Registrations have not fully lived up to expectations. In fact, they have remained flat during the past several years, and product experience reporting has even *decreased* substantially. This is an unsettling trend, one that I hope will be reversed."

Dr. Hayes wasn't in the FDA when the industry promised to voluntarily list its ingredients on cosmetic packages. Before it became mandatory, so few labels listed ingredients that finding one that did was akin to finding the proverbial needle in the haystack.

Dr. Hayes left through the revolving door marked "FDA Commissioners" in 1983, with the "unsettling trend" not likely to be reversed. If anything, the mandatory labeling regulation has proved that *no regulation can succeed on volunteerism because no regulation exists.*

Drug & Cosmetic Industry's editor Don Davis said of the remaining voluntary regulations: "All those things that, to me, make sense, and I'm sure, to the consumer, make sense, should have been made mandatory. A lot of people in industry obviously admit that they should have been made mandatory.

"If I'm going to report my plant or feel compelled to voluntarily report my plant and my adverse reactions, why shouldn't the plant across the street do the same thing?

"It makes no sense at all for someone to do it voluntarily who doesn't have to; especially if there's going to be some retribution or some FDA action that may affect me and not the guy across the street. When the FDA inspector comes and makes out an adverse report, you can't say 'Look at that guy across the street. He's dumping garbage out the window.' You can't say that. It doesn't work. He doesn't care about that plant across the street. There's a quota they're filling and he may not get to that plant.

"It makes no sense at all. It should have been made mandatory."

Ironically, during the pre-election Eagleton Hearings on Senator Thomas E. Eagleton's proposed cosmetic safety amendment to the Food, Drug, and Cosmetic Act, the CTFA, objecting to the premarket testing proposals in the bill, as well as in a number of other pending bills, claimed that CTFA had no objection to making the voluntary regulations mandatory.

However, there was a big "if." Since the CTFA had tailored its own voluntary program with its own safety net, it volunteered that "we would have no objection if the present Voluntary Program were made mandatory with provisions for continuing existing safeguards concerning confidential submissions."

The FDA could have picked up on the statement, gone ahead and made the voluntary remnants mandatory, and then attacked the industry-protective clauses. It could have acted as the regulatory agency taxpayers have a right to expect. It didn't.

As for the Eagleton bill, it went into the hopper to await another election year. When it emerged, it had been shorn of any effective premarket testing, and it was passed by the Senate as its members rushed out to attend to their reelections. The bill then disappeared into limbo and was never heard of again.

In October 1983, I was reminded by CTFA's president, Ed Kavanaugh, of CTFA's nonobjection to making the voluntary program mandatory; but in 1983, the cosmetic corner of the FDA, surviving on seven tenths of one percent of the FDA budget and under the administration's whip of "deregulation," was still writing speeches complaining about insufficient industry volunteerism.

Although the FDA in Washington failed to make company and product registration mandatory, one state did. As of October 1982, every cosmetic manufacturing facility in Florida must register annually with the state's Department of Health and Rehabilitative Services. Permits must be obtained to conduct business in the state and fees paid for the permits as well as for each new "separate and distinct" finished cosmetic product bearing a label with a Florida address.

CTFA representatives traveled to Florida to present their objections and recommendations; but the state prevailed where Washington failed.

QUESTIONS AND ANSWERS

If I write to the FDA, can I find out the ingredients used in a fragrance that has caused an allergic reaction or injury?

Not likely. If the cosmetic formulator has volunteered that information to the FDA, the FDA has been sworn not to reveal it. A better bet would be to have your doctor write to the company; but even then, the company is not required to reveal the fragrance ingredients unless it wants to.

If I were a little company and I wanted to do my own thing without letting the FDA know so that I wouldn't be bothered, wouldn't it be stupid of me to invite trouble by volunteering even that I exist to the FDA?

Apparently, a lot of people in the trade would agree.

Why did the FDA agree to clutter up its files with a lot of stuff when it's not likely companies are going to volunteer anything that might incriminate them?

At the time of the hearings, FDA claimed it couldn't implement the regulations because of its low funding. Instead of asking for sufficient funding, it elected to pass. The agency appears content to keep the cosmetic program so impoverished that it is literally dependent on the multibillion-dollar cosmetic industry for informational handouts.

Is Professor Page's Lawyering in the Public Interest still monitoring cosmetic regulation or nonregulation for consumers?

Unfortunately for consumers, we've lost our legal watchdogs on the steps of Washington where they count.

Now that Florida has shown that mandatory registration of cosmetic manufacturers and their products is feasible, couldn't Washington take the cue and do the same?

It could, but probably won't, unless you and a lot of others who care about what you put in and on your bodies and those of your family badger Washington into it.

‾ 11 ‾
Allergies and Injuries

It has been estimated that approximately fifty
percent of Americans are allergic to something.
—Harry Swartz, M.D.,
Author of *How to Master Your Allergy*

Adverse reactions take many forms. Allergies and allergens account for only some of them. Sensitizers can cause a previously nonallergic person to suffer reactions to the sensitizing ingredient whenever that ingredient is used in any product that comes in contact with the sensitized person. When the sensitizer is undisclosed, as it can be if it is a flavor, fragrance, trade secret, or used in trace amounts, choosing a nonreactive cosmetic is akin to playing a milder form of Russian Roulette.

An example of an unidentified sensitizer is 6-methylcoumarin (6-MC) which is a photosensitizer, activated by sunlight. Yet 6-MC was added to some of the most widely used sunscreens as an unlisted fragrance ingredient. The reported reactions to 6-MC went beyond what FDA termed "the usual transitory skin effects often associated with cosmetic allergic relations." In addition to reddening and rashes, blistering and systemic effects, some of which required hospitalization, were reported for years before products containing 6-MC were recalled. For every complaint that reaches the manufacturer or the FDA, countless others are never reported.

In asking for the recall of suntan products containing 6-MC, the FDA stressed that the reactions, mild or serious, could "lead to a chronic condition in which a sensitized person can have a skin reaction simply by being exposed to sunlight."

Although the recall was limited to sunscreens, FDA's cosmetic division director, Heinz J. Eiermann, later added, "Of course, also of concern have been the elicitation of photoallergic reactions and 6-MC uses in other types of products. A sensitized person may also suffer an allergic reaction from occasional use of, perhaps, a 6-MC-containing facial lotion." He might have added that photosensitization also can result in permanent discoloration of the skin.

The FDA, in its Washington perch, admitted it did not know how many people were allergic to the ingredient at the time, but claimed the agency was "particularly concerned because people not now allergic to 6-methylcoumarin may become sensitized to it if they apply it to their skin and then are exposed to sunlight."

After repeatedly announcing that it was proposing a ban on the use of 6-MC in cosmetics, FDA relegated the proposal to the dead-proposal bin along with the festering remains of proposals gone before.

Consumers who had products around with the sensitizer and who, until then, had escaped reactions still had no way of knowing which bottle might harbor the trick to be avoided.

Sensitization may occur with the first application, but sensitization is just the preliminary to a reaction. A subsequent reaction can occur with the next application. Both are unpredictable and can become manifest at any time ... even after repeated applications have not resulted in an adverse reaction.

Then, too, supposedly recalled products have been found years later on store shelves. When products containing hexachlorophene were recalled, I found a popular shave cream with hexachlorophene still being sold in some stores five years after the recall. Since hexachlorophene had been promoted as "good for you" before it turned out to be a killer, it was headlined on the package, so that the informed consumer could have avoided buying it. In the case of 6-MC, even the informed consumer was left with a shell game. As a legally unlisted fragrance ingredient, nobody had to tell and, apparently, no one has volunteered to tell.

Formaldehyde is a sensitizer of another sort as well as an irritant. It has been used in nail products almost as long as there have been nail polishes and bases and, more recently, in nail hardeners. It is also used as a preservative in cosmetics including shampoos, hair conditioners and rinses, liquid bubble baths, and mouthwashes.

Formaldehyde resins and formaldehyde combinations, used in certain nail-polish bases and nail strengtheners, have been known to penetrate the nails and cause severe dermatitis under the nails, to cause nails to become ridged, discolored, loosened, and to fall off, to cause pockets of fluid to form under the nails, to cause pain, disfigurement, and lawsuits to be won—but formaldehyde continues to be used.

On a rare occasion when an FDA cosmetic division staff member made an appearance at a consumer conference, Heinz Eiermann told a Washington conference on "The Future of Formaldehyde in Consumer Products," sponsored by the Consumer Federation of America, "The agency has not objected to the use of HCHO [formaldehyde] in nail hardeners provided the product (1) contains no more than 5 percent HCHO, (2) provides the user with nail shields which restrict application to the nail tip, (3) furnishes adequate directions for safe use, and (4) warns the consumer about the consequences of misuse and the potential for causing allergic reactions in already sensitized users."

For a number of years, the FDA and others have been conducting various tests and studies on formaldehyde. Patch tests done on patients in clinics throughout the world found that formaldehyde ranked among the ten most prominent contact sensitizers. In an inhalation study on laboratory animals, the Chemical Industry Institute of Toxicology found that, at fifteen parts per million, some rats developed nasal tumors, described as "squamous cell carcinomas."

Division Director Eiermann explained that the FDA saw no need to take any action on the use of formaldehyde since it claimed the cancers were localized, and epidemiological studies involving embalmers apparently did not produce the same results, although he did not discuss the studies or the results.

Even so, in some European countries formaldehyde is not permitted to be used in cosmetics, and it is possible to buy unformaldehyded nail polishes. In the United States, the so-called "hypo-allergenic" nail polishes seem to get along without formaldehyde. However, it must be remembered that the "hypo-" prefix only indicates a lower risk of allergy. There are no known non-allergenic cosmetics.

According to Mr. Eiermann, formaldehyde "is an excellent preservative" against unfriendly microorganisms such as pseudomonas aeruginosa, a pathogenic bacteria so virulent it can blind without warning within twenty-four hours. As an example, Mr. Eiermann cited a recent recall of almost half a million bottles of baby shampoo that was contaminated with pseudomonas and other microorganisms. According to the director, the problem arose when the manufacturer switched from formaldehyde to another preservative. However, the April 20, 1983 FDA announcement of the recall by Pennex Products Company, Inc. of Verona, Pennsylvania, stated: "The company has suspended use of the equipment thought to be the source of the contamination."

Certainly, formaldehyde has been known to be a good preservative over the years. The mortuaries have proved that. But there are other effective preservatives that have proved that all cosmetics do not have to be embalmed with formaldehyde. There is also the question of shelf life and use time, which neither the FDA nor the cosmetic industry has been willing to address. Cosmetics are not forever. There are expiration dates on perishable food and drugs; why not on cosmetics?

Contamination is one of the most serious, persistent, and widespread problems in cosmetics. It also presents one of the most serious risks to the general population, young and old, healthy or ailing—all are susceptible to the dangerous bacteria that can invade many categories of cosmetic products. Unfortunately, because of the lack of adequate inspections and sanitation controls, some cosmetics are contaminated before they reach the market.

When half a million bottles of baby shampoo are recalled from the stores, there may be a like number already in the homes and nurseries. The Pennex recall also illustrated how one private-label company can blanket the country and appear under multiple labels, yet still be the same shampoo.

According to the FDA, the Pennex baby shampoo was sold under more than two dozen house brands and was "contaminated by bacteria that could infect scratched or cut skin or scratched eyes." It was distributed nationally under its brands,

Soothex and Mara Lynne, and under Pennex's generic label (called simply "Baby Shampoo"). It was also distributed as the Treasury brand baby shampoo by the Treasury Drug Division of J. C. Penney Company, and as the Army and Air Force Exchange Service's AAFES Baby Shampoo as well as under a variety of house brands.

Heinz Eiermann said, "Cosmetics need not be sterile; however, they must not be contaminated with microorganisms which may be pathogenic, and the density of non-pathogenic microorganisms should be low to prevent spoilage which may be harmful. In addition, cosmetics should remain in this condition during their use by consumers.

"The hazard of inadequately preserved cosmetics to human health has been amply demonstrated by reports of staphylococcal infections in hospitals from use of contaminated creams and lotions."

With the problems that have occurred with contamination of cosmetic products routinely used on infants and the hospitalized, it may be advisable *to require those products to be sterile*. Cosmetic staples, such as talcum powder, baby oil, shampoo, cleansers, and lotions, are more routinely used than are drugs on infants who have yet to develop an immunity to any unfriendly bacteria as well as to a "density" of what the FDA considers nonthreatening bacteria. Since those staples also are used in hospitals on infants and on patients whose immunity is decreased or nonexistent, it seems eminently reasonable to require sterility of those products.

Mr. Eiermann failed to explain that infections were mysteriously happening in hospitals when it was discovered that not only the topical preparations being used on patients, but the hand lotion used by nurses just *handling* patients, were found to be contaminated with bacteria that were causing the outbreak.

In one test, all samples of a hand lotion, opened and unopened, were contaminated with a variety of virulent microbes ranging from 44,000 to 7,500,000 microorganisms per milliliter. So, after another "recall" (which is never a recall of all the products found in the stores, hospitals, and homes), it was business as usual again. And those same product categories have continued to be found to be contaminated *again* and *again* and *again*.

Mascara and eye makeup is another category that repeatedly has been found to be contaminated with the very bacteria, *pseudomonas aeruginosa,* that can attack a scratched eyeball and result in blindness. Scratching an eyeball is not as difficult as it may sound when mascara is hurriedly applied with a brush that has picked up the bacteria from a tube of contaminated mascara. It happened to a college student who suffered excruciating pain before being blinded. For her, time and nature mercifully thinned the corneal scars. After a year of blindness, the victim was fitted with special contact lenses, and she was able to regain at least some of her sight. Chemical analysis of the mascara showed that the preservative broke down at temperatures between sixty-five and seventy-five degrees and allowed the dangerous pseudomonas bacteria to develop.

According to Dr. William J. Evans, who was with the FDA's Bureau of Drugs, "Pseudomonas infection is highly resistant to therapy. The literature reports approximately a hundred cases of pseudomonal infection of the cornea resulting in loss of the eye. Statistically speaking, this figure is but the top of the iceberg.

"The wider use of contact lenses, particularly by women, and the frequent occurrence of at least microscopic abrasions, may increase this hazard a hundredfold. But rare in occurrence or not, it is not in any way justified if it is preventable. Statistics are a poor answer for the victim in whom the results have been 100 percent hazardous."

When the industry and the FDA admitted that the problem went beyond isolated cases, they had an interesting solution. They took a published report on corneal ulcers that had been linked to contaminated mascaras and used it to recommend that consumers discard mascaras after a short period of time to prevent using contaminated mascaras.

In 1980, the FDA said it had documented sixteen cases of corneal ulceration and thirty-two less serious cases of eye infections associated with the use of mascaras contaminated with high counts of bacteria or fungi. Pseudomonas organisms were implicated in most cases of corneal ulceration. When the contaminant is *pseudomonas aeruginosa,* and the cornea is accidentally injured with the applicator brush, the FDA said, "the infection may cause ulceration which can lead to partial or total blindness in the injured eye."

Investigations showed that "poorly preserved mascaras pose a serious hazard to health," and the FDA claimed, "The mascaras become contaminated with microorganisms during repeated normal use." The agency also volunteered that it thought most manufacturers had "reevaluated their preservative systems" and improved the effectiveness. Besides, it said, the highly contaminated mascaras implicated in the corneal ulceration had been withdrawn from the market.

But again, even a cosmetics watcher had no way of knowing which of the mascaras already in use might hold the threat of blindness.

Back in 1977, the FDA, "responding to the mascara-contamination problem," published one of its impotent proposals. This one was supposed to require that cosmetics coming in contact with the eye "contain preservative systems that effectively protect them against microbial contamination during normal use."

The agency solicited information on testing standards and procedures that could be used to check the preservative's effectiveness in use. Apparently, the industry that takes inordinate pride in voluntary self-regulation did not rush to provide the methodology, because, according to the FDA, "No useful information was received." Consequently, the University of California in San Francisco was given a contract to come up with the "required methodology and standards."

"Meanwhile," said the FDA, it had not "ruled out regulatory action to remove from the market those products that injure the eye as a result of inadequate preservation and, thus, contamination." It was a regulation that already existed and had since 1938 when "Cosmetics" was made the weak sister of the Food, Drug, and Cosmetic Act.

Years later, nothing has been heard of the methodology or of further safeguards to "respond" to the "mascara-contamination problem."

However, the industry did rush to alert its consumers to discard their mascara tubes quickly before the mascara was used up to avoid contaminating their brushes, which could damage their eyes if a brush should scratch them. The discards, of course, should be replaced promptly with newly purchased (by the consumers) mascaras. Beauty editors and columnists picked up the cry and, crazily, the onus and responsibility of a safe and serviceable product was transferred to the consumer at the consumer's expense and the producer's profit.

Nowhere was it suggested that it might matter how long a tube of mascara may have been on the store shelf before the consumer bought it and how well that preservative system was holding up. Nowhere was it suggested that if the manufacturers were concerned with their preservative systems not being adequate to the expected use of the entire product, the product might be packaged in smaller sizes. Since many companies have had promotions of mascaras in trial sizes or with recurring "gift with purchase" offers, why not make the smaller sizes regularly available so they could be used up faster and possibly prevent contamination? If cosmetic companies were reluctant to give up the higher price for each purchase, they could package two of the smaller sizes together and, thereby, split the odds for contamination. Also, until a methodology surfaces for insuring safety throughout normal use, dating packages is a serviceable idea.

No one will argue the importance of eyes that see. Unfortunately, even the keenest eyes cannot see what may be lurking in a half-used tube of mascara.

To quote Dr. Evans, the hazard "is not in any way justified if it is preventable."

QUESTIONS AND ANSWERS

Which Pennex baby shampoos were recalled?

The recalled lots of Pennex baby shampoo distributed nationally under its brands Soothex and Mara Lynne, and under Pennex's generic label (called simply "Baby Shampoo"), were listed by FDA as: A13F, A17F, A28F, D20E2, F14E, F16E, G13E, G14E, G14E1, G22E, G29E, H12E, H13E, H16E, H18E, H19E, H24E, H24E1, I1E, J4E, J5E1, J5E2, J6E, J6E1, J8E, J8E1, J12E, J20E, J20E1, J21E, J22E, J25E, J25E1, K22E, K30E, L1E, L3E, L6E, L6E1, L7E, L13E, and L20E.

The shampoo also was distributed as the Treasury brand baby shampoo by J. C. Penney's Treasury Drug Division, and as the Army and Air Force Exchange Service's AAFES Baby Shampoo, as well as under the following house brands:

IN THE NORTHEAST:

Baby-Mate, distributed by Adams Drug Co., Pawtucket, R.I.

Courtesy, distributed by Port Washington Distributor, Port Washington, N.Y.

Drug Guild, distributed by Drug Guild Distributors, Secaucus, N.J.

Filene's, distributed by Filene's Sons Co., Boston, Mass.

Happy Harry's, distributed by Merchandisers, Inc., Newark, N.J.

Heck's, distributed by Tri-State Distributors, Inc., Nitro, W. Va.

LSA, distributed by L. S. Amster & Co., Inc., Westbury, N.Y.

Medalist, distributed by Spectro, Jenkintown, Pa.

Tops, distributed by Niagara Frontier Services, Buffalo, N.Y.

Top Value, distributed by S&P Drug, Brooklyn, N.Y.

West Medical, distributed by West Medical, Inc., Framingham, Mass.

IN THE SOUTH:
Kerr, distributed by Kerr Discount Drug Stores, Raleigh, N.C.

Our Brand, distributed by SAS Products, Jacksonville, Fla.

Rose's, distributed by Rose's Stores, Henderson, N.C.

Shopper's Drug Mart, distributed by Shopper's Drug Mart Inc., Boca Raton, Fla.

IN THE MIDWEST:
Baby Touch, distributed by B and E Sales Co., Detroit, Mich.

Coop, distributed by Universal Cooperatives, Minneapolis, Minn.

Elder-Beerman, distributed by Elder-Beerman Stores, Dayton, Ohio

Gold Circle, distributed by Gold Circle Division of Federated Stores, Worthington, Ohio

Seaway, distributed by Seaway Foods, Cleveland, Ohio

Sunfresh, distributed by Sunfresh Inc., St. Paul, Minn.

IN THE WEST:
F&D, Benicia, Calif.

What is the best way to apply eye makeup?

Carefully and unhurriedly. Ignore the quickie makeups sometimes promoted on beauty pages to publicize skilled makeup artists. The two-minute complete makeup is not for the unhandy when it comes to applying mascara safely or artistically—no matter which "easy-do" mascara wand is being promoted.

When applying mascara, brush the lashes with mascara away from the eyes without getting too close to the eyes. For definition of the eyes, use an eyeliner and shadow first and concentrate the mascara on the outer edges of the lashes. Keep the eyeliner muted in tone, whether using a soft pencil or liquid. Some prefer to soften or to clean the line with a cotton-tipped swab or to finger-smudge the liner. By keeping the liner muted and the mascara away from the rims of the eyes, most eyes look larger instead of caged in with heavy or dark outlines.

Most important of all, use a magnifying mirror in a bright light. If you wear glasses, put them on after you've made up and check your eye makeup. Clean up the mistakes with a clean, soft, and flexible cotton-tipped swab dampened with water or hand lotion, depending on the solubility of the makeup.

Since there is so much emphasis on eyes and eye makeup, what can be done to give eyes definition in a hurry if mascara is not used?

Stay with an eyeliner and a bit of eye shadow. Some eyes even look better without mascara. Try it.

If you're lucky enough to have dark, lustrous lashes, treasure them and show them off. It beats covering them up with mascara and trying to keep the lashes separated. Keep them soft and glowing with a tiny bit of petroleum jelly or castor oil. It's the look the cosmetic industry has been trying to reproduce with chemicals and alchemy.

If contact lenses are worn, should some precautions be taken when using eye makeup?

Indeed. Many ophthalmologists advise their patients to forego mascara when wearing contact lenses and warn against using the nonwater-soluble mascaras, which usually are described as being "waterproof" or "twenty-four hour" mascaras.

As Dr. Evans cautioned, there's a possibility of microscopic abrasions of the cornea, which can be infected with contaminated mascara and cause injury. Flakes of nonwater-soluble mascara also may contribute to the abrasions if they come between the contact lens and the eye.

If mascara must be used, be sure it's water-soluble. Buy only well-sealed packages of the smallest sizes from a store with a fast product turnover. Don't buy refills for the brushes unless you intend to thoroughly clean and sterilize the brush before using the refill—even so, it's not worth the trouble—and keep all your makeup fresh and clean. *All* makeup or anything else that might come near or in contact with the eyes should be fresh and clean.

12
Babies...What You Don't Know Can Hurt Them

The problem today is not so much the products
that are known to harm, but the cosmetics that
are not known to be safe.
—Winton B. Rankin,
Former FDA Assistant Commissioner

If further proof is needed that cosmetics go beyond powder and paint, all we need do is watch a mother returning from the hospital with her newborn infant. Most likely, she's returning with a promotional kit of baby products. Among the samplers may be talcum powder, baby oil, a lotion, a cream, a cleanser, and perhaps even a baby shampoo and bubble bath—all qualifying as cosmetics.

In using cosmetics intended for infants and young children, it is prudent to remember that infants, in particular, do not have the same natural defenses against unfriendly bacteria and questionable substances that people acquire later in life.

At the earliest age, the child, without the adult defenses, shares the risks of allergic reactions, sensitization, and outright harm from misunderstood cosmetic practices, misinformation, and cosmetics that are presumed to be safe but may, in fact, not have been sufficiently tested to be judged safe. Since cosmetic products are not required to be tested or cleared for safety or purity before they are marketed, extra caution should be taken in buying and using any cosmetic product intended for babies.

"Medicated" on a label may appear to be adding a bonus to the product. The added drug or chemical, however, may not only be unneeded but may present a hazard.

Hexachlorophene is a prime example of a heavily advertised and promoted ingredient that pervaded so many grooming products for years before it was relegated to prescription-only status.

Although the safety of the disinfectant had been questioned for nearly a decade when it was found to be easily absorbed through the skin and to have caused systemic damage, injuries, and deaths, the FDA did not act to curtail the generalized use of hexachlorophene until after some forty babies had died after being dusted with talcum powder containing 6 percent hexachlorophene.

On September 27, 1972, the FDA ordered the immediate recall of products containing more than 0.75 percent hexachlorophene. Infant powders were singled out for special concern because they were applied repeatedly, were not rinsed off, and were covered by diapers.

The FDA recall and ban came two days after *The Wall Street Journal* reported on a University of Washington study that showed brain damage had occurred among newborn infants who had been routinely washed with hexachlorophene solutions.

Boric acid, purported to be a sure killer of cockroaches, can be indiscriminately lethal. Infant deaths have been reported from what some have claimed to be the misuse of potentially toxic boric acid and boric acid products.

However, *The Merck Index,* the encyclopedia for

chemists, pharmacists, physicians, and members of allied professions, claims that death has occurred from less than five grams of boric acid in infants and from five to twenty grams in adults.

The classic reference work lists various uses for boric acid, ranging from weatherproofing wood, fireproofing fabrics, and hardening steel to cosmetics. Medically, it has been used topically as a bactericide and fungicide. The *Index* also notes:

> *Human Toxicity:* Ingestion or absorption may cause nausea, vomiting, diarrhea, abdominal cramps, erythematous lesions on skin and mucous membranes, circulatory collapse, tachycardia, cyanosis, delirium, convulsions, coma.

> —Chronic use may cause borism (dry skin, eruptions, gastric disturbances).

> *Caution: Several cases of fatal poisoning have occurred following its absorption from granulating wounds and abraded skin areas.*

Cosmetic chemist Gabriel Barnett, writing in *Cosmetics, Science and Technology,* examined the controversial use of boric acid in talcum powder. One study "emphasized that boric acid is added to the talcum powder primarily because it is one of the most practical buffering agents for this purpose, and not as an antiseptic."

Nevertheless, Mr. Barnett observed that boric acid had been replaced by other buffer systems in some baby powders. He noted that, "After consideration of the many differing reports, opinions, and official pronouncements, some pediatricians still do not recommend the use of boric acid in baby powders, lotions, and ointments. This ingredient has been deleted from some baby powders partly for commercial reasons and possibly for medical reasons."

Mr. Barnett characterized pure talc as one of the most

useful toiletries for babies, adding that pure talc without any additives is preferable. Medication, if needed, should be left to the decision of a physician.

Regulators in other countries apparently agree with Mr. Barnett. Japan, for one, has banned the use of boric acid in all talcum powders.

In *The Medicine Show,* the editors of *Consumer Reports* cautioned against the use of medicated powders for diaper rash, noting that there is no proof that the commercially available powders help prevent the rash. Furthermore, "Since baby powders with antiseptics sensitize the skin of some infants, they should be avoided, as should soaps with antiseptics, unless prescribed by the baby's doctor."

Mr. Barnett also cited medical warnings that "antiseptic" oils may cause sensitization and noted the preference for sterile mineral oil.

From within the industry, Mr. Barnett inadvertently has touched on the nature of "baby oil." "Baby oil," as it is bought and used for practically everything from oiling babies to oiling suntans, is basically perfumed mineral oil. For a fragrance, which may or may not be a sensitizer or an allergen, consumers are paying many times what they would pay for pure mineral oil that serves the same purpose with less risk for sensitization or allergic reactions. Any mother will tell you that bathed babies smell sweet without adding an alien fragrance or other cosmetic ingredient that increases cost as well as risks.

Apart from subjecting infants and toddlers to the risks of sensitization and allergy, toiletries promoted for children have caused irritation, pain, and injury. Notably, bubble bath products aimed at children, as well as those for adults, have a history of injuries. Despite the accumulation of medical and consumer reports and FDA studies confirming the adverse reactions and injuries, industry representatives have succeeded in not only resisting adding a warning statement on the product labels, but apparently convincing the FDA to go along.

On January 28, 1977, the FDA published its proposal for a label warning on bubble bath products. The warning statement was intended to caution consumers against product misuse and to recommend discontinuance of use and consultation with a physician should injury occur.

As background to its *Federal Register* proposal, the agency said it had received many complaints from consumers and physicians about adverse reactions caused by bubble bath products. "They reported itching and skin rashes; urinary tract, bladder and kidney injuries; and genital disorders. Other persons reported eye irritation and respiratory disorders. A significant number of injuries required medical attention."

The FDA cited medical reports of injuries attributed to detergents in bubble bath products as far back as 1955. In 1965, S. Marshall reported in a *Journal of Urology* article, "The Effect of Bubble Bath on the Urinary Tract," a case of urinary frequency, urgency, and painful or difficult urination in a two-and-a-half-year-old boy. The condition disappeared when bubble baths were discontinued.

In 1966, H. N. Bass, in a *Clinical Pediatrics* article, " 'Bubble Bath' as an Irritant to the Urinary Tract of Children," described four cases of genitourinary tract injuries in children. The injuries were associated with bubble baths and were representative of a total of sixteen children with urethral and bladder irritation attributable to the use of bubble bath preparations. The symptoms ceased or were alleviated when the use of bubble baths were stopped.

Although the ingredients causing the reported injuries could not be definitely determined by the FDA, the available information indicated that the source of the adverse reactions appeared to be alkylarylsulfonate. According to the agency,

"Alkylarylsulfonates are general purpose detergent and wetting agents for use in industrial, household, and cosmetic products. Some alkylarylsulfonates have been widely used in all types of bubble bath products as detergent and foaming agents. The skin defattening and irritation properties of detergents are widely known."

In 1971, the FDA contacted "all cosmetic firms known to manufacture bubble bath products" with the request that the industrial detergent be reduced to less than 10 percent of the formulations or, preferably, between a 2- and 5-percent concentration; and to remove all other harsh ingredients. The firms were also asked to monitor the frequency and types of adverse reactions "because a safe concentration of alkylarylsulfonate had not been determined and additional reduction or elimination of the detergent ingredient might be necessary."

The FDA admitted that its request to the bubble-bath producers did not significantly change the number of consumer complaints during the ensuing years. In fact, in 1973, when the Federal Trade Commission became concerned enough about the problem to solicit consumer reports of adverse reactions to bubble baths in the Cleveland, Ohio area through the press and radio, FDA received sixty reports of adverse reactions. In a six-month period that prompted the FTC action, FTC had received twenty-nine complaints at its Cleveland office. The FDA had received thirty-seven complaints from its various offices, but had taken no action.

In its 1977 label warning proposal, the FDA admitted that the combined FTC-FDA "data further indicate that many adverse reactions may be expected to remain unreported unless consumers are encouraged to report their experiences; even then, many consumer injuries may not be brought to the attention of FDA."

Unaddressed is the fact that many injured or uninjured consumers have no way of knowing that the *Food* and *Drug* Administration also is the agency for cosmetics. Few can be expected to know where to complain if injured or beset with adverse reactions, since the "cosmetic program" is hidden in the Bureau of Foods. Since bubble bath or other cosmetics are neither *food* nor *drug*, where does one go to complain?

Even if a letter finds its way to the FDA, what can be expected? As an investigative reporter specializing in cosmetics for twenty-five years, I asked one of my prime sources in the FDA about the current status of some color additives. I was referred to another department. I also was assured that, if I wrote and requested the information, it would be forwarded to me without delay. I followed precise instructions in requesting readily available material, identified myself as a writer with a deadline in two months, and addressed it to the head man with his mail code so that the letter would not stray. Two months later, I had received neither the requested material nor an acknowledgment of my letter.

In its long-winded apologia in proposing a simple warning statement from the industry, the FDA went through its "tabulations and analyses of the reports" the agency had received and decided they showed "that many commercial bubble bath products have caused adverse reactions. The greatest number of complaints is related to the leading children's bubble bath product. The second highest number of complaints is associated with another [unidentified] widely distributed children's product.

"The majority of injuries and the most severe injuries, i.e., genitourinary tract disorders were reported in children, particularly female children."

All this wind-up began with reports kept from 1967— ten years before the FDA published its mild proposal and *twenty-two years* after the publication of a medical report of the problem.

The FDA then covered pages with descriptions of how the detergents used in the bubble baths were removing protective sebum from the skin's surface and extracting lipids from the cell membranes of the skin's outer layer. It told of the resulting dry skin and how the increased friction of dry skin on dry skin "may cause itching, redness, chapping, or fissuring of the skin, and in severe cases may induce inflammation and infection. Mucous membranes may undergo similar changes leading to irritation, inflammation, or infection. In severe cases of mucosal damage and microbial attack, urogenital tract infection may occur."

Finally, "Because of the many reported adverse reactions to bubble bath products, the commissioner intends to make these requirements effective 6 months after publication of the final regulation in the *Federal Register*. The time period between publication of the final regulation and the effective date of the regulation should provide adequate time to make the required label changes. Accordingly, the labels of all products initially introduced into the interstate commerce 6 months after publication of the final regulation must bear adequate directions for safe use and the required caution statements."

The label proposed for bubble baths was to bear adequate directions for safe use and the following caution:

CAUTION—*Use only as directed. Excessive use or prolonged exposure may cause irritation to skin and urinary tract. Discontinue use if rash, redness or itching occur. Consult your physician if irritation persists. Keep out of the reach of children.*
    In the case of products intended for use by children, the phrase *"except under adult supervision"* may be added at the end of the last sentence in the caution required . . .
    In the case of powder products, the phrase *"Avoid inha-*

lation of dust to prevent respiratory discomfort" shall be added to the last sentence . . .

Six months later, labels had not changed. Industry representatives objected to the language, the definition . . . protested that things were not that bad that any warnings were needed—and the proposed regulation was stayed.

On August 19, 1980, the FDA made another attempt at a label warning on bubble baths. There was a new commissioner and a more forceful brief for the proposed labeling.

Eighty-two comments had been received by the agency during the comment period of the 1977 proposal. Sixty-five fully supported the proposed warning, two supported it but requested exemptions or modification, and five opposed it. Ten comments were neutral, some proposing a ban on bubble bath products. Three comments received after the expiration of the extended comment period fully supported the labeling proposal.

Industry objections were voiced primarily by The Cosmetic, Toiletry and Fragrance Association, which was successful in getting a month's extension on the comment period. The CTFA was also successful in narrowing the definition of bubble bath products to exclude spreading oils which contained a surfactant and not the cleansing detergents and foam stabilizers of other bath oils which would remain in the definition. Also, the inhalation warning was downplayed because FDA was assured that offending powdered preparations had been reformulated. However, the request for at least a two-year delay in the effective date of this "final rule" was rejected. FDA thought a year was enough time to reprint labels.

"Such a delay would be contrary to FDA's mission of effective consumer protection," said the FDA in its changed voice. The effective date for label warnings on bubble baths introduced in interstate commerce would remain, as proposed, August 19, 1981.

The proposal, signed by then Commissioner Jere E. Goyan, effectively answered the objections and concluded: "FDA advises that the human experience information received from consumers, physicians, and the industry fully supports the conclusion that the proposed label warning on bubble bath products is needed to reduce the risk of future harm."

Among the comments supporting the caution were those from five physicians who told of bubble bath preparations causing many cases of urinary tract infection in children. Some children had undergone unnecessary, expensive urological evaluations for cystitis, only to have their symptoms abate when they stopped using the bubble bath products.

The FDA pointed to the five comments as supporting its findings discussed in its 1977 proposal "that bubble bath products can cause adverse reactions, particularly when misused, as when consumers use excessive amounts of bubble bath, take bubble baths too frequently, or remain in the bath for a long period of time, thereby subjecting themselves to prolonged exposures to a product."

That should have done it, but in 1981, there was still another commissioner and a new president. CTFA's Political Action Committee also had been very active during the 1980 election. The climate had changed in Washington and the consumers had been put in deep freeze.

Two months before the "final rule" for bubble bath warnings was to become effective, the restructured FDA sent out a press release. On June 1, 1981, the FDA announced it intended "to stay temporarily the effective date of a rule requiring that bubble bath labels use cautionary labeling that prolonged use may cause skin or urinary tract irritation."

In 1983, under the 1981 commissioner replacement who, himself, was about to be replaced, the *Federal Register* published a regurgitation of the proposals dating back to 1977, noting that, on April 17, 1981, The Cosmetic, Toiletry and Fragrance Association petitioned the FDA "to revoke the bubble bath label caution requirement and, while FDA considered the merits of this petition, stay the effective date of the regulation."

The CTFA repeated the objections that had been effectively overruled by Commissioner Jere Goyan in the pre-election months of 1980. This time, it also pointed to the post-Reagan-election "administration policy" that "supports a stay and withdrawal of the regulation in question, which places an unnecessary burden on industry." (See Chapter 8.)

So, on February 18, 1983, the "temporary" stay of June 1, 1981, became the proposal that all regulation relating to bubble bath products "be stayed pending a final decision on this proposal." The proposal was signed by FDA Commissioner Arthur Hull Hayes, Jr., who resigned shortly after its publication.

All this over a simple warning to consumers to use bubble bath products with care to avoid risks that, with a warning statement, could be easily avoided . . . *risks that were known to exist for almost thirty years.*

Through it all, a letter written by the father of an injured child to the Office of Consumer Affairs echoes and re-echoes. The Office of Consumer Affairs had received a flood of complaints about bubble baths, but it's doubtful that the complaints were counted with those received by the FDA or FTC. The letter was representative of many in the office's thick file.

The father wrote:

> About the first of January 1970, my wife put a little more than a cup full of a [children's bubble bath] product into our boy's bath.

> The product produced burns or excessive irritation around the most vital body area of the child. For three-four days he was in *crying pain.*
>
> I was furious as any father would be and wrote to the [manufacturer]. The reply I received was fairly apologetic, but it really did not answer my question which was: Why can't the whole box, if spilled by a child, be used and cause no side effects—except for allergy-affected people? Our child was not allergic to any products at this time.
>
> The product *should* be able to be put into the bath without causing any burning or irritation . . .

Indeed, with all the years of rhetoric, the father's valid question was not addressed: *Why can't the whole box, if spilled by a child, be used and cause no ill effects?*

It's no wonder that, early in the industry-agency tug of war, *Drug & Cosmetic Industry* Editor Don Davis tagged it "The Bubble Bath Caper." Don Davis also introduced an interesting sidelight. During the early 1970s, when the complaints were heaviest among the children bubble bathers, he told of private meetings of the CTFA (then called TGA) and the FDA, after which CTFA asked its members to "consider taking out the suspected irritating ingredient from their bubble baths. There were no recalls or seizures by the FDA, and the market was still filled with children's bubble baths the agency no longer considered safe.

The FDA did issue two formal complaints: one to the Gold Seal Company, better known for its Glass Wax, producer of Mr. Bubble; and the other to the Purex Company, better known for its laundry bleach, producer of Bubble Club Fun Bath. Both companies were outside the cosmetic industry community. Neither was a member of the trade association.

In an editorial, titled "Peculiar Goings-on," Mr. Davis examined the "outsider" aspect of the two companies. According to Mr. Davis, the trade association had argued persuasively for its members; and since the two noncosmetic companies were "unlikely to have the cosmetic scientific resources to refute the arguments in the FDA complaint without weeks or even months of outside laboratory work," the companies apparently had found it more expedient to agree to reformulate their products.

Mr. Davis concluded: "It can teach many in the industry a valuable lesson that routine testing of many products intended for use by children may not be enough. A product that gives a child pleasure is an invitation to overuse, and overuse is bound to turn up peculiar manifestations not producible through normal skin irritations, eye sensitivity, or hair damage studies. Such peculiarities as this urinary tract irritation will only turn up in three-month or six-month use studies. The message seems to be that at least in some products, overtesting is mandatory."

Apparently the "outsiders" also have capitulated to voluntarily putting warning statements on the labels of bubble baths intended for children. The stock of bubble bath products examined on store shelves shows that Mr. Bubble and other "fun" bubble bath products for children have added a cautionary warning. Most of the other bubble baths, one of which was labeled as being for the entire family, had no cautionary statements.

During an interview with Ed Kavanaugh, CTFA's president, I asked him about the long-term controversy, noting that the FDA was still getting quite a few complaints from consumers about bubble baths.

"Couldn't you just say to your members, 'Hey, let's do it. It's not a big deal,' and end that?"

To expend that much time and energy, as well as the money, for twenty years over a simple warning seemed insupportable.

"Well," Mr. Kavanaugh told me, "we have to reflect, at CTFA, what our members want. They're our clients. We have to discuss with them and try to lead them in the right direction. They feel strongly that those products are safe if used as directed . . . and they don't feel that this product should be singled out if it is abused."

However, in the case of products intended for children, I told him I thought the father whose youngster was injured by bubble bath was reasonable when he asked: *Why can't the whole box, if spilled by a child, be used and cause no ill effects?*

"Doesn't that make sense to you?" I asked Mr. Kavanaugh.

"Well," he said, "I guess in an ideal sense it would be. I don't know what the answer is."

When I had failed to get a concession from Mr. Kavanaugh that the bubble bath vendetta could be ended, he acknowledged that there were some areas where he wished the FDA would be stronger. He declined to specify the areas, but explained, "I think when there is an abuse out there . . . if the government would step in once in a while and say no, that would keep things in line. And I think, sometimes, the government has to do that.

"A more decisive FDA is what we need . . . more decisive in making tough decisions . . . instead of sitting back and doing nothing."

QUESTIONS AND ANSWERS

What is a baby's best protection when it comes to using the necessary toiletries?

A careful mother with access to a good physician when necessary.

Is boric acid still being added to baby powders?

Yes, in some. Check the labels—especially those that claim the powder is "medicated."

Is it advisable to use any medicated toiletry on babies?

Caution and many pediatricians reject the use of any medication unless there is a condition that requires medication, and then a physician should be consulted.

Is it possible that some of the rashes may be a result of prior sensitizations from scented or medicated baby products that have been used?

Yes, but your doctor would be the most likely person to know. Check your baby and all the products you've used with the doctor and follow his advice.

Would you recommend using any bubble bath for babies or young children?

No. Mild soap and water does the job.

What would you suggest to make baths for babies and children more agreeable than merely necessary?

Tender loving care from the mother and maybe wrapping the baby or young child in a warm fluffy towel after the bath. One of my earliest memories is of my mother wrapping me after a bath in a large bath towel that she had warmed, taking me in her arms, and tucking me into bed. Taking a bath was a treat that netted me the warmed towel and a frothy hot chocolate before bedtime as I grew older.

Babies are not born with a yen for bubble baths. Why fall for the commercial brainwashing?

— 13 —
Teens and Other People

Teenagers represent a $20 billion market that is a
growth industry.
—**Seventeen Magazine**

Not long ago, when girls in protected circumstances
were told they looked "sexy," it might bring a blush and, perhaps, even an attempt to flatten a readier-than-most emerging
bosom. But that was before the cosmetic and jeans industries
got together and decided that teens were marketable and profitable, and sexy was in.

By 1980, even the late teens were out and what used to
pass for teens was pushed to tens as ten-year-old nymphets
came in. Suddenly ten- and twelve-year-old girls were made up
to look like twenty-two-year-old sex objects in provocative
poses. Photographers claimed they didn't have to contend with
wrinkles that had to be retouched. Apparently, by concentrating on preteens, they also avoided dealing with acne.

With the advent of nymphets, makeup artists became
celebrities. To go along with the little-girl-into-siren phenome-

non, there were dolls and doll heads, complete with makeup kits to paint dolly's face and ersatz dye to change the color of dolly's hair. There were makeup kits for the preteenager and for the near-infant . . . learning tools for the present and future consumers of sexy jeans and elaborate makeups. Between the two industries, their exploits covered both ends. Cherubic cheeks, painted and denimed, greeted everyone everywhere from every medium.

Since, with time, even the tens become teens, the cosmetic industry has seen to it that there are no awkward ages in cosmetics. Lines, such as Tinkerbell cosmetics for kids, bridge the gap between childhood and teenhood. Little girls can choose flavored lip gloss before graduating to adult lipsticks without ever baring their lips.

Yet, with all the flaunting of the young, the teen years remain years of insecurities, of self-doubt, of striving to match the painted and denimed ideal.

The selling of the very young and more-than-beautiful fantasy has effectively put many, if not most, teenagers in a vise. Even the most beautiful can wonder if perhaps the color of her hair is wrong. After all, Clairol *does* sponsor a number of programs aimed at the young . . . and look at all those Plain Janes transformed into sirens with flowing blond hair. Maybe blonds *do* have more fun.

Left unsaid in the glamorous commercials and advertising is the fact that the producers of the artificial hair color take their cue from every color and shade of young or teenage hair. It is in those tender years, before the hair is subjected to harsh cosmetic measures, that hair is considered to be at its vibrant best. In attempting to create believable color, the producers of hair dyes seek the ideal of capturing not only the color but also the natural sheen and subtle tones of a teenager's hair. The ideal has yet to be reached.

Practically any attractive, and even a beauteous, female can be transformed into dowdiness simply by changing her hair style, dress, and her expression as well as makeup. Conversely, almost any Plain Jane can be transformed into seductiveness with the help of a talented makeup artist, a skilled hairdresser, and a $2,000 designer gown ... *without changing the color of her hair.*

A fairer "before and after" demonstration would be to use the same model with the same transformation—with and without the changed hair color—and allow the viewer to make the choice. Nature has been known to make mistakes, but not many.

In courting the young, the cosmetic industry capitalizes on the inherent insecurities endured by both sexes during adolescence. Young men are courted by role-model sportsmen hawking everything from shampoo and after shave to acne preparations. Shaving has become the battleground of before-, during-, and after-shave products as well as the shavers and their blades.

Both sexes were courted by Pat Boone, once a teenager's singing idol, and now the father of Debbie Boone, who inherited the mantle.

Charles E. "Pat" Boone became the president of Cooga Mooga, Inc., of Los Angeles, and spokesman for Acne-Statin, an acne "treatment" produced by Karr Preventative Medical Products (KPMP) of Beverly Hills, and sold through the mail for almost ten dollars. As the principle spokesman for Acne-Statin, Pat Boone appeared in print and on television enthusiastically endorsing the "treatment."

The Federal Trade Commission, which in 1978 was checking advertising more closely than in more recent years, decided that a celebrity's recommendation was not enough to substantiate the advertised claims. Consequently, the agency issued a complaint against Karr Preventative Medical Products and Atida H. Karr, M.D., charging that false and unsubstantiated claims were made for Acne-Statin.

In part, FTC's complaint against KPMP and Dr. Karr alleged:

> Acne-Statin neither will cure acne nor can eliminate its cause, as claimed; they have falsely advertised that Acne-Statin is superior to all other acne preparations and to soap in the antibacterial treatment of acne; contrary to other claims, there are time and quantity limitations on the money-back guarantee for Acne-Statin; and there was no reasonable basis for claims that Acne-Statin will cure acne and result in skin free of acne blemishes, or for various other performance claims.

In signing the consent order for himself and Cooga Mooga, Inc., Mr. Boone agreed that he and Cooga Mooga "must have a reasonable basis when making any claim relating to the efficacy, performance, any characteristic or property, or the result of use of any product. Also, they must make a reasonable inquiry into the truthfulness of any proposed endorsement of this nature."

Mr. Boone also agreed to pay "his pro rata share of any restitution which might be ordered by the Commission or by a court." Later, Mr. Boone filed an appeal to review his agreement to pay the restitution. On October 3, 1983, however, the case was resolved with Mr. Boone ordered to pay his pro rata share of twenty-five cents on each bottle of Acne-Statin on which a refund was authorized. According to the FTC, Mr. Boone's final obligation of $5,591.50 was satisfied when Dr. Karr of Karr Preventative Medical Products deducted the amount from certain money owed to Mr. Boone.

Among other things, the consent agreement prohibited misrepresentations of

> the benefits Boone family members have derived from any product; product tests or product test results; and the efficacy, use or

performance of any product where the use or misuse could affect the user's health and safety.*

Although dermatologists are seeing an increasing number of older adults with acnelike eruptions being attributed to the use of cosmetics, adolescents remain the most vulnerable to cosmetic medication claims. Teenagers, plagued with acne at a time when social acceptance is crucial to them, are prime targets for any new product offering salvation from the plague. Too often, teen-aimed advertising offers more than the cosmetics can deliver.

For an occasional blemish, some over-the-counter acne preparations can be helpful. However, when they are classified as cosmetics and therefore escape required testing, they may contain ingredients that have been found to be photosensitizers. In some persons, a reaction to sunlight or a sunlamp could result in replacing the spots they hope to lose with spots that are not easily lost.

Until there is greater assurance that the products can help without harming, it would be prudent to check acne products and their ingredients with a family doctor or with the FDA. Best of all, a visit to a dermatologist at the onset of acne or any skin eruptions most likely will prove to be the most effective and least costly.

If, however, you feel your problem is minor enough for you to treat, a recent report by the Advisory Review Panel on Over-The-Counter Antimicrobial Drug Products may help in checking the ingredients in a product before buying it.

* Note: The consent agreement entered into by Mr. Boone and Cooga Mooga, Inc. is for settlement purposes only and does not constitute an admission by them that they have violated the law. When issued by the Commission on a final basis, a consent order carries the force of law with respect to future actions. A violation of such an order may result in a civil penalty up to $10,000 per violation being imposed on a respondent.

The panel reported that acne sufferers could successfully treat themselves with nonprescription lotions, creams and gels containing sulfur, benzolyl peroxide, or sulfur combined with resorcinol. Sulfur and benzolyl peroxide were judged safe and effective for treating acne and preventing new acne lesions when used separately, as was the sulfur combined with resorcinol. However, since benzolyl peroxide and sulfur both are skin irritants, products that include the two ingredients together should be available only on prescription and used carefully according to a doctor's instructions.

According to the report, acne affects about 80 percent of all adolescents and some older persons as well. It cannot be cured, but it can be successfully treated with properly constituted nonprescription drugs by more than three-fourths of the people suffering from it. It should be noted that the doctors who participated in this report were referring to *drugs*, which are more strictly controlled than cosmetics. Even so, some severe cases of acne require prescription drugs under the supervision of a physician.

In reviewing the ingredients in over-the-counter acne products, the panel found that benzolyl peroxide or sulfur alone reduces lesions and continuous use will reduce the development of new lesions. Sulfur combined with resorcinol or resorcinol monoacetate also was found to be effective, but resorcinol alone was not effective.

Although abrasive scrub products are useful to wash oily secretions of the skin and to keep pores open, these products have no beneficial effect on acne lesions.

QUESTIONS AND ANSWERS

I am sixteen years old and a junior in high school. I have medium brown hair and am wondering if I should dye it red or bleach it blond. I keep hearing commercials that tell me coloring the hair is good for it. Can you advise me?

At sixteen, your hair, if regularly washed and brushed and left alone, is at its best. Dyeing or "coloring" or bleaching the hair definitely is not "good" for it, no matter what the commercials say.

A change of color might improve a person's appearance or even help someone who's older, or whose hair is prematurely gray, overcome the prevailing prejudice against older people in getting a job. However, at sixteen, your hair—or hair like yours—is providing the inspiration for the colorists in their attempt to reproduce the colors, shine, and highlights that youth and good health endow you with naturally, without charge, and without your having to spend hours with the dye pot.

If you check the boxes of hair color, you'll probably find your color glamorized as "golden," "sunlit," or "moonlit" brown. Enjoy the real thing while you have it. Accept no substitute until and unless you have to.

There are products on the market that look like scouring pads that are supposed to slough off dead skin. Are these recommended for teenage skin?

Not if you have breakouts or a sensitive skin. Plain soap and water usually is the best "treatment" for adolescent skin.

Does makeup harm the skin?

It shouldn't, but it doesn't help it either. Young skin is fresh and envied by those who no longer have it and spend fortunes in an attempt to recapture it. If you must wear makeup, try to avoid covering your skin with foundations or powder unless it's a medicated foundation prescribed by your doctor to correct or alleviate a condition. You're better off with lip gloss and a little eye makeup, skillfully applied, on special occasions. Otherwise, learn to appreciate the glow you now have that commercial makeup tries to mimic.

What's the best way to be attractive while growing up?

Becoming addicted to cleanliness. There's nothing more appealing than having an aura of scrubbed cleanliness. That means daily baths or showers, shining clean hair, clean and unbitten nails, immaculate grooming, and fresh, clean clothes, no matter what your style.

‾ 14 ‾
Men's Day

The big cosmetic companies aren't into eye
shadow for men yet, but New York males who
want it get it anyway.
—Town & Country

In a bravura prediction of the future, *Town & Country,* the magazine for and about socialites, predicted makeup for men and tossed off the claim that men already were dipping into women's makeup as well as enjoying special products "just for the strong sex like face bronzers, gel, glow sticks, and cover tones."

In 1971, when *Town & Country* was marking its 125th anniversary, literal makeup for men might have seemed likely. Some men were turning up with their faces covered with "bronzers" that made them look jaundiced, mottled terra cotta, or muddy brown. A hot day found some of them reporting for work streaked with rivulets that trickled the "bronzer" down to their collars and ruined their shirts.

For a while, practically every cosmetic company was

rushing to create new lines for men. Most simply repackaged cosmetics originally intended for women, replaced the feminine scent with musk, and sailed the "new" breakthrough for men into the marketplace. Elizabeth Arden was able to come up with twenty "Arden for Men" cosmetic items, and packed ten in a travel kit with the suggestion that the kit could later become a sewing box.

Revlon brought out a number of cosmetic lines for men, among them "Pub," which featured "Below the Belt Deodorant Spray ... a deodorizing men's powder spray for the groin area."

It was a time of television commercials that costarred men with cosmetics. There was the handsome male who rose out of bed and boasted that he had not used his antiperspirant yesterday and might not use it today ... and the viewer was left to wonder if that was why he was sleeping alone. A man's cologne that might have made a companion piece to the commercial was called "Sweat," not to mention the one called "Balls."

Another burly male confessed to using baby powder to keep cool and still another to washing his hair with baby shampoo. A well-known comedian vowed he'd "never be gray again" as he demonstrated a metallic "color restorer" on his hair, only to be seen being "gray again" in the following years.

Newspaper and magazine advertising featured more esoteric cosmetics such as special lotions that ranged from after-shave moisturizers and hand lotions to wind-sun-cold-weather lotions and a wrinkle-smoothing lotion. There were toners and moisturizers, gels and creams, and lip pomades.

The bath or shower became a ritual with bubbles and foams and soap on a rope. There were after-bath or -shower body lotions, moisturizers, splashes, or talcum powder. Deodorants and antiperspirants came in colognes and toilet waters as well as the many usual forms.

Hair, always a focal point for sales, became bigger business as "color restorers" vied with "hair color (never say dye) for men"; beauty salons became unisex, and fancy shops had "men only" nights. Barbers became "hair stylists" and raised their prices accordingly. The "blow-dry" became part of standard vocabulary. There was a choice of permanents for men, and hair sprays—all of which made all kinds of hairdressing and conditioners necessary. Toupees became "hairpieces," and hair was attempted to be put back where there was none by transplanting and by a number of other ways. Through barbershop windows, men could be seen having face masques, and elite skin salons advertised their facial care for males.

And, of course, there were those bronzers, glow sticks, and green talc to tone down "ruddiness."

Everyone seemed to be getting into the male act, including the Europeans with, especially, the French companies elbowing the Americans. It was a carnival of times.

The courting of the male had found its impetus in the mid-1960s when those in the cosmetic industry decided it was time to sell more fragrance to men even though, in total gallonage, men were already using more fragrance than women.

In a *Drug & Cosmetic Industry* article, "Too Much—Too Soon in Men's Toiletries," Peter Vautin counted thirty new lines of men's toiletries that had been introduced in three months. He warned that the fragrance market, in particular, had become top-heavy. In addition to being "swamped by a rush of newcomers ... practically every French perfumer and treatment house almost simultaneously offered a new men's line." Furthermore, "established companies" had introduced second brands with a full line of products.

Peter Vautin's prophecy has been borne out by the sagging sales in fragrance in the 1980s despite the continuing launching of more and more lines of fragrances with designer names and price tags.

In the 1980s, the carnival is over. Apparently, there is makeup for men as *Town & Country* predicted, but it is being used not by its socialite readers but by those in the punk bands and culture who have espoused the outrageous in their own calculated carnival of times.

Still, there are enough designer colognes and after-shaves for men in phallic-shaped bottles and enough "toiletry kits" that sprout on Father's Day and at Christmastime for women to buy for men. Some men buy their own, but it will take some doing before eye shadow for men will be a big seller.

Some male "treatment" products are still treated to generous advertising budgets by potential *Town & Country* advertisers such as Estée Lauder and various clothing designers who lend their names to cosmetic labels for a price reflected in the price tag.

Apart from the elitest offerings, men continue to contribute their share to the sales of cosmetics. Most men use toothpaste, shampoo, a whole range of shaving products, deodorants, and a medicine cabinet full of other cosmetic-toiletries. They also share the risks and benefits of the cosmetics they use, along with the women and children.

However, men have retained an advantage in what is now referred to as a gender gap. Although the bulk of the dollars come from women who are bombarded with manipulative advertising and psychologically high-priced cosmetics, women have practically no representation among those who hold the reins of the cosmetic industry, its administration and regulation.

Since the passing of Helena Rubinstein and Elizabeth Arden, a strong feminine hand is missing at the top, despite the feminine names that have found fame on cosmetic labels. Any industry meeting of executives, cosmetic chemists, or those involved in research and development ... any visit to Washington and the "cosmetic program" ... any contact with legislators or regulators ... will find you in man's land.

Check your local agency; see if you can get beyond the female "public affairs officer," "consumer affairs officer," or whatever the publicity woman may be called. If you succeed, ask a question that is logical for a woman consumer to ask and experience the chauvinism of the male who probably won't know what you're talking about, doesn't care to know, and most likely will dismiss you as being a troublesome crank.

Often, only if injury or tragedy touches home will action be taken. Many a regulation happens as the present cautionary statement on cleaning products happened—after a legislator's child swallowed a bleach and there were no instructions on the label as what to do about it.

Sometimes, a comic-tragedy among males will net females an action that had been indicated for years with adverse reactions in females. Take, for example, the Canadian banning of estrogenic hormones in cosmetics.

For decades, it has been known that estrogenic hormones in cosmetic formulations are not enough to show any practical benefit to the skin but enough, if uncontrolled, to cause systemic changes. Among the changes are abnormal bleeding in females, sex changes in males, and premature and/or abnormal sex changes in children who had dipped into Mommy's hormone cream. Also, estrogenic hormones have been known to cause cancer in animals.

Estrogenic hormones are *drugs;* and as the late Dr. Stephen Rothman, who was professor emeritus of dermatology at the University of Chicago, told a group of cosmetic chemists: "There is no drug which sooner or later would not cause any harm if given without any restriction of the dosage; if it can be given without limitation, it is not a drug. It cannot be denied that in the case of cosmetics which are applied once or several times daily and often on relatively large surfaces the amount absorbed and permitted to have systemic effects is entirely uncontrolled."

One doctor told of a hysterectomy that had been performed on a menopausal woman before it was learned that the abnormal bleeding that had led the woman to seek medical help might have been traced to her use of twice the amount of an estrogenic cream and lotion that the FDA had determined to be safe.

The agency had determined that the use of two ounces of a product containing 10,000 international units of estrogens per ounce, over a thirty-day period, would normally not cause systemic changes. However, at the time and for years after, Helena Rubinstein was packaging "hormone twins" in sales promotions that included an oil and a cream, both containing 10,000 units of estrogens, and nowhere was the purchaser informed that to use both simultaneously was to double the amount considered to be safe.

The doctor concluded: "Continuous absorption of small doses of estrogens over a long period of time can produce endometrial hyperplasia [excessive cell growth and subsequent shedding of the inner lining of the womb] ... If estrogen creams continue to be sold over the counter without prescription, it should be mandatory that [they carry] a label bearing a warning advising intermittent and not continuous use as well as a statement recommending a limitation of quantity to be used."

Another woman in her mid-thirties bought a hormone hand lotion on sale and used it, as she had used her usual lotion, after almost every hand washing and over most of her body after every bath. For the first time in her life, she found herself bleeding between menstrual periods. She had seen enough posters citing abnormal bleeding as one of the first signs of cancer to report to a cancer clinic. The first examination proved inconclusive and she was told that perhaps there was a blister that might have to be removed. Since her mother had died from cancer after an operation, she delayed returning to the clinic.

In the meantime, she finished the bottle of hormone hand lotion and replaced it with her usual nonhormone lotion. She had not been questioned about cosmetics during her examination, so it was accidental that she didn't buy a second bottle of the hormone lotion. The abnormal bleeding ceased and, when she returned for an annual checkup, no abnormality was found.

Later, she learned of hormonal absorption through the skin and possible systemic effects. Her delay in returning to the clinic may have saved her from a needless operation.

Children also have been victims sharing the hazards of indiscriminate use of hormones in cosmetics. Because consumers are uninformed and unaware that hormone cosmetics are not merely cosmetics but are as much drugs, though less potent, as the birth-control pills sold only on prescription, children and hormone creams, in particular, have been mixing with alarming results. Numerous premature and abnormal sexual changes in children caused by the ingestion of various hormone cosmetics have been reported.

One three-year-old girl with a six-month history of breast enlargement, accelerated growth in height, and vaginal bleeding, was brought to a hospital by her worried mother. According to the doctors: "Repetitive and insistent questioning . . . disclosed that the child periodically played with and ingested a discarded dermatological preparation containing 10,000 units of estrogen per ounce. Withdrawal of this product promptly caused regression of the laboratory and clinical changes."

The doctors warned: "These findings indicated that dermatological preparations widely held to contain insignificant quantities of estrogens represent a significant and unrecognized environmental health hazard to the pediatric age group."

When the FDA decided on the 20,000-unit-per-month safe limit, most of the over-the-counter hormone creams contained 10,000 units of estrogen per ounce. Labeling, however, did not then and does not now give adequate instructions for use, nor have any been found to advise that use be limited to one product to keep within the thought-to-be-safe limit.

Despite more than forty years of acknowledging that estrogens could be absorbed through the skin and cause systemic changes—that they did cause cancer in animals and might stimulate the growth of existing tumors—and clinical studies that showed no discernible improvement in the skin beyond that of the base cream without the estrogens, hormone cosmetics were allowed to continue undisturbed until January 1, 1978.

As of January 1, 1978, Canada prohibited the use in cosmetics of "estrogenic substances which recent scientific studies have shown to be potentially carcinogenic."

The news of the impending ban was dropped casually by R. B. Smyth of Canada's Health Protection Agency during a 1977 conference in Brussels on International Cosmetic Regulations.

In the preceding years, the Canadian Broadcasting Corporation had televised a number of programs on cosmetics and cosmetic safety, focusing, among other aspects, on the questionable use of estrogenic hormones in cosmetics. When reminded of the programs, Mr. Smyth said his office had received many letters from women questioning the safety of estrogens in cosmetics. However, he added, they had been waiting for documented proof of harm. This they had, according to Mr. Smyth, after a man went to a barbershop and discussed the sparsity of hair on his chest with his barber. The barber suggested that a bottle of lotion containing estrogenic hormones be rubbed on his chest. The entire bottle was applied in one operation.

Instead of the expected hair on his chest, the barber's client developed what appeared to be rudimentary breasts, a change of voice, and impotency. As he sought medical attention, the Canadian Health Protection Agency apparently found its documentation for banning estrogenic hormones in cosmetics to be sold in Canada.

According to Mr. Smyth, the Canadian authorities felt that there was no need for risk in a cosmetic product when there were other ingredients available to cosmetic manufacturers.

Later, Michael Alexander, Canada's Health and Welfare information officer, questioned "that the regulation was promulgated in response to any particular case or testimony." His explanation: "Estrogenic substances were prohibited in cosmetics because of scientific evidence that estrogens could be absorbed percutaneously; and because of statistical evidence that continued exposure to estrogenic substances could give rise to endometrial carcinoma."

Meanwhile, back in the United States, ingredient listing in the order of predominance knocked out the necessity to specify the number of units of estrogenic hormones contained in an ounce of cream, lotion, or liquid. The precautionary guidelines, recommended by the FDA, became meaningless since even well-informed consumers had no way of knowing how to keep within the no-more-than-20,000 units of estrogens per month.

Despite FDA in the United States not following Canada's

lead, the Canadian ban may have been noted by U.S. companies who send their products across the border. Estrogens have disappeared from the labels of all but a very few creams and lotions for women.

Instead, lesser-known companies have turned to the men and are luring them with hormone-containing products for the hair—or lack of hair. Some of these products are labeled "hair food"—a term that would have sent the FDA on the run a number of years ago when the very term would have qualified for mislabeling.

One "hair success treatment" listed an unspecified amount of "Estrogenic Hormone" midway in its list of ingredients. The labeling described the product as "a fine blend of Hormones, Amino Acids, Protein, and Vitamin E. For damaged, breaking hair; hair that doesn't grow." It neglects to tell the hopeful user what "success" to expect from the "treatment." Neither does it warn that the product contains an active drug, set limits for application, or caution to keep it out of the reach of children.

In examining a shelf of hair products, from tonics to pomades, containing estrogens and apparently aimed at balding men, I found that none had an indication that it was other than cosmetic. Questions to the cosmetic division of the FDA were fielded to the Division of Drugs. No one questioned seemed aware of the Canadian ban or of the "hair foods."

Finally, there were no answers as to why, amid all the warnings being given on hormone prescription drugs that are medically prescribed and supervised for a relatively modest percentage of the population, nothing is said of over-the-counter hormone cosmetics hawked to the general population without warnings—and without any proven efficacy beyond what the hormoneless base might accomplish.

Could it be that there are men who are experiencing the

symptoms evidenced in Canada but are not aware that what they're rubbing on their scalps might be affecting other parts of their bodies? Without a warning against overuse, how would a possible victim be expected to know? Without the specified quantity of estrogens contained in a jar, how would *anyone* be able to judge what would be *overuse*?

Women's insecurities, which have been so well programmed by the cosmetic industry, are matched by the sensitivity of men whose hairlines have begun to slip. The sensitivity has been made more acute with the advent of television where every male facing the camera seems to have the hair he had when he was nineteen.

At sixty-two, the Hollywood actor making a personal appearance for his latest movie is brought forth with a well-covered scalp and only slightly graying hair. Few on-camera males have either attained the security or have been allowed to keep their own hair or lack of it as it is.

Even the smooth heads of Kojak and the king of Siam are seldom reprieved. Those who are pictured as being sparse of hair have been relegated to second-banana or character roles, untouched by romance. Is it any wonder that the balding male is ripe for the advertised magic potions that are "guaranteed" to grow hair or to prevent baldness?

In 1980, the promotion of "baldness cures" became so flagrant that the FDA "proposed to remove from the market products claiming to grow hair or prevent baldness."

The agency acted after an expert advisory panel reported that no products sold to grow hair or prevent baldness are effective. If the proposal becomes final, a manufacturer who later discovered an effective drug to grow hair or to prevent baldness would have to provide the FDA with proof of its safety and effectiveness before it could be legally sold.

According to the panel, the most common type of baldness occurs in men over an extended period of time and is an inherited trait, as are hair color, texture, and curliness.

Hair loss also can result from malnutrition produced by crash dieting, an iron deficiency, a hormone imbalance, or exposure to radiation. A sudden excessive hair loss or an unusual pattern of hair loss may have an underlying medical cause. The panel recommended that anyone having such a problem consult a doctor promptly.

"Nothing done to the hair shaft once it emerges from the surface of the scalp will influence hair growth," the panel advised. "To demonstrate that an ingredient is a hair restorer, it must be proven that the active ingredient gets to the hair root and stimulates hair growth.

"Sex hormones taken internally can stimulate hair growth but the growth of hair may not be in the desired places. These hormones, available only by a doctor's prescription, are not recommended for retarding baldness.

"Applying hormone-containing products to the scalp and hair won't have any effect on hair growth unless large amounts are applied for a long time." However, the panel warned, "such excessive amounts applied to the hair and scalp can cause male breasts to enlarge."

Other than the hormone "hair foods," the panel found that the "baldness cures" they examined contained ingredients such as lanolin, olive oil, wheat germ oil, and vitamins—none of which will grow hair or prevent baldness.

Nothing more has been heard of this, yet another FDA proposal. But the announcement was made before a certain elder President with a full head of dark hair took office. Since then, the "baldness cures" have continued to flourish unabated.

In another sphere of covering the male head in particular, the reported injuries and horrendous results could not continue to be ignored. On June 3, 1983, the FDA banned the sale of artificial hair fibers for scalp implantation "to ensure that the dangerous practice of implanting these fibers in bald heads is not revived."

The ban applies to fibers of such synthetic materials as polyester, modacrylic, and polyacrylic, and also to some natural materials, such as human hair processed for implantation on another head. It does not apply to natural hair transplants in which a person's own scalp hair and surrounding tissue are grafted to another part of the scalp.

The technique usually consisted of implanting hundreds to thousands of synthetic fibers at a cost of thousands of dollars. The process took two or three days and usually was not done by physicians. According to the FDA: "Contrary to advertising claims, the fibers were not effective either in simulating natural hair or concealing baldness. Within a short time after implantation, the fibers usually fell out, broke off, or were rejected by the body."

In March 1979, the FDA issued a public warning about the implants. An FDA nationwide investigation resulted in several regulatory actions including three administrative detentions and four seizures. The FTC and several states also took some actions against firms.

From December 1978 through February 1981, the FDA received 166 complaints and the FTC received 181. Injuries included infection, facial swelling, severe pain, scarring, and permanent loss of the victim's remaining real hair. Many required extensive medical and surgical treatment. In seven cases, surgical removal of portions of the scalp was necessary. In twenty-one cases, the fibers could not be removed and the patients' scalps remained disfigured.

In its investigation, the FDA found that *no* currently available type of hair fibers or synthetic hair-implanting technique is safe or effective. If anyone is able to develop safe fibers, the FDA said the manufacturer could apply and the ban would not preclude their approval. As far as is known, no one has yet come up with a safe and effective way to either grow or implant hair other than that produced by the host subject himself.

QUESTIONS AND ANSWERS

Lately, I've noticed a red rash on my face that seems to flare up particularly after shaving. I've used the same shave cream and after shave for many years, and I've never had any reaction.

Naturally, if any product is suspected of giving you a reaction other than the one you intended, the best thing to do is to stop using it and see if the reaction subsides.

Although you may have been buying the same products, the formula may have been changed. Unless you can find out what your past purchases contained, you've no way of knowing whether one or more ingredients have been changed or even the ratios of ingredients or process. A note to the company responsible for the products might give you an answer.

Often, the cosmetic ingredients may be innocuous, but the fragrance, which doesn't have to be identified, is the offender in causing allergic reaction—or even sensitizing a person who previously has not been allergic. Subsequent exposure to that ingredient may result in an allergic reaction to other products containing the ingredient.

My hands get chapped in the winter. Is it all right to use the same hand lotion my wife uses?

Chapped skin is chapped skin. If the fragrance of your wife's hand lotion doesn't disturb you, then use it. When the big push was on to sell two products to men and women, the only change made in most was to change the fragrance and the packaging. Check the ingredients and you'll find them basically the same. Water heads them all, then mineral oil or glycerin, some form of lanolin, or a variation that acts as an emollient or a humectant. Contrary to the old saw about water and oil not mixing, the cosmetic industry has found a way to mix water and oil with various emulsifiers.

Do you have any advice for the man who is self-conscious about being bald or having less hair than he'd like?

If lack of hair really bothers you, there's always the instant cure for baldness—a hairpiece—but you might be just as self-conscious about wearing one.

Unless there is a medical problem that is causing hair loss, your genes are the most likely programmer of your hair. Check your doctor for any medical reasons. Don't fool around with cosmetic come-ons. Once you know there is no medical reason for the hair loss, get to love your genes for all the other qualities you've inherited.

Best advice: You're much more than the hair on your head. Some men have made careers from having high foreheads or smooth heads. Good grooming and a firm, healthy body, character, and a sense of humor count much more than a full head of hair. By the time your hair has left you, you should have developed into a more interesting person than when, in retrospect, you were a callow youth with a full head of hair. If you haven't—get to work becoming one.

What about the hormone "hair foods"?

You can wash it, oil it, curl it, dye it; but you can't feed hair through its ends. It must be fed through the bloodstream by the same food that feeds the rest of your body. Maybe that's why someone long ago thought to call the other ends of our hair "roots." Like the plants that depend on their roots, which, in turn, depend on whatever they get from the soil and environment, human hair depends on whatever is being given and whatever is being done to the rest of the body.

Ever try feeding the petals of a rose after it has bloomed to force it to grow more petals?

15
The Body

Treat it kindly. It's the only body you'll ever have.
—Toni Stabile

During a consumers' conference on cosmetics sponsored by a community college, an overweight, balding representative from the cosmetic industry ran some slides of beautiful, slim, nude and seminude women to illustrate the benefits of cosmetics. Among the women used to illustrate these benefits of cosmetics was Raquel Welch, whose body obviously was not the result of cosmetics.

The audience hooted as the representative tried to convince the unconvinced that the products manufactured by his industry had worked the magic that produced the likes of Raquel Welch. Unfortunately, the industry had sent a representative who, while having ready access to all the magic of the cosmetic industry, was not the male equivalent of Raquel Welch. Nature may have bared his head, but the gentleman remained responsible for the rest of his body.

When asked why only women's bodies were bared and displayed although the industry also sold cosmetics to men, he answered that the male body was not as attractive to look at as the female body. The response was: "It depends on who's looking at it." It might have been, "It also depends on the shape it's in." A well-formed body is beautiful no matter what the sex. Any art gallery has evidence of physical beauty created and existing long before Rubinstein, Arden, and Revlon.

Ancient Egyptian sculptures and paintings of Nefertiti show her to have been of exquisite beauty. Although the sculptures and paintings of her head are the most renowned, it is only when her entire figure is seen that her extraordinary beauty can be fully appreciated.

Although the ideal body measures eight heads tall, and the average body measures seven heads, the cosmetic industry seemingly chooses to ignore the fact that the head is only a fraction of the whole and that skin, hair, and nails go with it.

Flashing a perfectly formed body, male or female, and relating it to a shampoo or the newest mascara or the latest moisturizer with the inference that you, too, can be thus if you buy this, is calculated bait for the gullible.

In the 1920s and early 1930s, before the Federal Trade Commission was given the power to regulate advertising that took advantage of consumers, the infant cosmetic industry offered those concerned about their weight magic "slimming creams" and bath salts that were advertised as being able to float fat down the drain. The products and claims disappeared when the FTC and FDA were empowered to monitor cosmetic advertising and labeling.

Decades later, "slimming cream" reappeared at an international cosmetic show in Bologna, Italy. Within a few more years, variations of "slimming creams" crossed the ocean to find their place on American store counters.

The reincarnation of the "slimming creams" may be traceable to the emergence of a new word in the unbeautiful-body vocabulary—*cellulite.* In *Webster's Unabridged Dictionary,* the closest to *cellulite* is *cellulitis,* which is defined as "an inflammation of a cellular tissue, especially of subcutaneous tissue." In the commerce of beauty, *cellulite* was advertised as something the French called " '*Peau d'orange*' (orange peel skin)—skin with bulges, ripples."

Dermatologists and other medical authorities claim "cellulite" is nothing more than fat under the skin that causes the skin to dimple and ripple. Lose the surplus fat, and you lose the ripple effect that the French, especially, have fancied up to introduce the new clones of the "slimming creams."

In 1978, Methode Elancyl Beauty Massage Regime Kit, Elancyl Gel, and Elancyl Bath Foam were recalled because the FDA charged that the products were being sold with false and misleading labeling. Elancyl is the brand name of those ubiquitous green packages of body products and the green-and-white massager shaped to fit around the hand.

If the FDA thought Elancyl overdid the labels, the moribund FTC apparently was looking the other way when, in 1982, Pierre Fabre, Inc. took three full-color pages in *The New York Times Magazine* to advertise the various Elancyl products.

One page was headlined: "DO YOU TRULY UNDERSTAND YOUR BREASTS AND HOW THEY KEEP THEIR SHAPE AND OFTEN DON'T?" Readers were then given an illustrated explanation of the breast and assured that if the Elancyl Beauty Solution and Cream were used "faithfully . . . you will have made a major step in helping your breasts keep (or actually improve) their shapely line and alluring appearance."

The opposite page was headlined: "YOUR HIPS AND THIGHS. IS THERE A WAY TO TAKE CARE OF WHAT THE FRENCH CALL

'CELLULITE'?" The ad was illustrated by the now-familiar slim, nude body with no trace of "cellulite," being soaped with the Elancyl Massage Glove.

Readers were assured "THE METHODE ELANCYL WORKS . . . And it isn't even a matter of losing weight. It is a matter of, perhaps, five minutes a day. If you are loyal, chances are you can lose up to an inch off your thighs in 3–4 weeks." The "Methode" included three products that were meant to work together on your hips, thighs, and buttocks.

Elancyl had competitors in the slimming-cream race. One, La Crème Body Contour Cream, offered results not in "3–4 weeks," but promised, "Lose Up to Two Inches From Those Problem Areas in Just One Hour."

In Bloomingdale's extensive cosmetic department, a stripling-slim company representative was selling La Crème at $30 a jar while a television monitor demonstrated how the cream was supposed to be liberally smeared on the body and then snugly wrapped in six or seven layers of plastic wrap. (The plastic wrap was not included, but a number of super-market brands were recommended.)

After the mummy-wrap, you were to pop yourself into a robe or get under a blanket and relax for an hour—*no more*. After you cut away the plastic wrap with blunt-point bandage scissors, La Crème would continue working away if you stayed slippery and didn't take a bath or shower for six to eight hours.

La Crème was not to be used on the breasts or face. This could mean learning to live with big breasts and a fat face while the rest of you got smaller. For those who might find wrapping themselves in six or seven layers of plastic tedious, La Crème also promised to be effective without the plastic wrap.

Without the plastic wrap, La Crème was to be used after a morning shower. Just "smooth the cream over your ab-domen, buttocks, hips, and thighs. Then carefully slip on panty hose or leotards, avoiding slippage of cream as much as possible. Go about your daily routine while the cream tones and conditions your skin."

Enough consumers thought it was too good to believe and turned to the FDA for confirmation that the FDA prepared a "Talk Paper" about La Crème. FDA Talk Papers are prepared by the Office of Public Affairs "to guide FDA personnel in responding with consistency and accuracy to questions from the public on subjects of current interest."

The September 11, 1981 talk paper informed the personnel that "A nationwide promotion is underway for La Crème, Inc., New York, N.Y. and Morristown, N.J. Advertisements claim that the product will 'help melt away inches of unwanted bulge in just 60 minutes.' "

The FDA talk paper revealed that ads, which apparently had floated by the FTC, also said that the cream's "gentle warmth penetrates deep into your skin and helps melt fatty deposits."

Word of the FDA surveillance may have reached La Crème, Inc. before the Bloomingdale's demonstration in 1982, which may account for the disclaimer on a printed sheet of instructions and the descriptive folder, both of which could be considered to be labeling and therefore in FDA territory. The disclaimer noted that La Crème was confined to shedding inches and not weight or fat.

According to the talk paper, "Promotional literature distributed to retail stores and franchises (though not necessarily to consumers) also claims that FDA has approved or classified La Crème as a skin toner, tightener and smoother."

Consumers and reporters who inquired about La Crème were to be advised:

No known product can penetrate the skin and melt away fat.

La Crème, the product, has not been reviewed, analyzed, or approved by FDA.

FDA has received neither safety-and-efficacy nor adverse reaction reports about La Crème. (Promoters claim La Crème's formulation was invented in California 12 years ago during arthritis research. The Bureaus of Drugs and Medical Devices and the Division of Cosmetics Technology have no record of any related correspondence.)

FDA is looking into La Crème's market status under the law. The firm claims La Crème is a cosmetic.

Any loss of inches due to combining a cream product with a body wrap probably is due to a transitory "wristwatch band" pressure effect which will disappear soon after the wrap is removed. Any loss of weight due to induced moisture loss will be regained as soon as the user eats or drinks.

The talk paper, which was a personnel briefing, did not become a news release. Left in ignorance, there apparently were enough hopeful gullibles to keep the "slimming creams" selling and more "body-wrap" franchises sprouting and flourishing throughout the country.

QUESTIONS AND ANSWERS

How should the body be treated?

Kindly and with consideration. Treat it as a whole and remember that how you feed, exercise, and use it is how it will respond. Educate yourself in proper nutrition and keeping the body healthy. Sleep is a magic wand. See that you get enough of it. Lots of water inside—drinking six to eight glasses of water a day—is the best moisturizer for your skin.

Cleanliness is paramount. Start with a clean body and then protect it from the elements—a good sunscreen to protect your skin from too much sun that will cause premature wrinkling and might invite skin cancer, and an all-purpose hand-and-body lotion to keep all your skin moist and protected.

Cosmetics have their place, but don't count on them to give you a model's body.

What about the body creams that are being advertised as tightening "spongy skin"?

I've yet to see human skin that looks like a sponge. I suspect that some copywriter, realizing that *cellulite* may have had a bad press, has come up with a substitute word. The plant-life ingredients—or "botanicals"—that are currently popular are almost identical to those spicing the "slimming creams," which still cling to using "cellulite" to sell to the uninformed, the I-don't-cares, or the gullibles.

Basically, any cream that creates a barrier between the moisture in your skin and the outside world serves the same purpose. Unless you intend to use the cream for massaging, or your skin is extremely dry, you will probably do best using lotion on the body.

What about massage creams and body massage?

Massage creams are designed to work with the massaging hands and the body they're massaging. Flesh is more easily manipulated when the skin is greased. The cream is then washed off. If it's not contaminated and there's nothing in it that can cause a reaction, it's a pleasant way of oiling the skin and keeping it supple.

A massage can be relaxing, but don't count on it to reduce you.

What about the allover body perfumed deodorant sprays?

Who needs them? They're certainly no substitute for soap and water, and a bath or shower takes care of all of you.

These are perfumed sprays that include a deodorizer, which in itself is a contradiction. Why take a chance on being sensitized to a fragrance all over your body—or risking an all-over allergic reaction if you happen to be allergic to an ingredient that, if part of the fragrance, is not identified?

An antiperspirant or deodorant used in the armpits would be more to the point. If you want to smell of perfume, use your favorite scent where it's not likely to surprise you with a breakout. When I use perfume or a perfume spray, I use it on my hair where the scent lasts and can't do much harm.

I enjoy taking bubble baths. How can I use the bubble baths in the market safely?

You can cut your odds of irritation from bubble baths by using half or less than half the amount suggested in the instructions and by not soaking in your bath for a long time.

16
Hair

Rapunzel, Rapunzel, let down your hair!
As soon as Rapunzel heard this, she took her long
braids, wound them once or twice around a hook
outside the window, and let them fall twenty ells
downward toward the ground. This made a ladder
for the witch to climb, and in that way she
reached the window at the top of the tower.
Rapunzel, Rapunzel, let down your hair.
The marvelous tresses were lowered at once. The
Prince climbed the silky golden ladder, and
stepped through the tiny window up above.
—Tales from Grimm,
translated by Wanda Gag

Although few, if any, can boast of having Rapunzel's silky golden hair, strong enough for witches and princes to climb, strong lustrous hair is eminently desired throughout the land. Billions of dollars are spent in its pursuit.

Entire magazines are devoted to the culture of hair. Other periodicals regularly allocate space to hair and how to wash, curl, uncurl, color, uncolor, condition, cut, style, groom, and grow it.

Bald barbers often are able to convince their balding clients that their new tonic will definitely grow hair where there is none.

Practically everyone has some kind of hair, and almost everyone is faced with the problem of what to do with it. And just about anyone is ready to tell or sell something about it or for it.

Hair is big business all around. The media serenade the sellers and the sellers reciprocate by advertising with large clumps of dollars.

Unfortunately, hair has become an object of abuse in the mad pursuit of what appears to be better on the other person's head. Never have there been so many "conditioners," even while the hair-dye commercials insist that the advertised product (which is bound to be heralded as "new and improved" within the month) will make your hair better and "feel soft around your neck."

The hair-dye manufacturers urge consumers to get into the dye pattern earlier and earlier. Gray is only a mean dictionary word. Silver is not mentioned except on package labels, which suggest that, if you insist on "going gray," your natural color must be covered with *steel* or whatever other term the copywriter created to edge away from the dreaded *gray*. There are also rinses "to take away the yellow"—those usually are seen on the blue- or lavender-haired women.

For those who have yet to worry about "going gray," there are beautiful young models who are shown as becoming "ravishing" with a new hair color ... and a new hairstyle and new makeup and an extravagantly expensive designer gown and, of course, new lighting—which is the biggest flatterer of all.

For the puberty set, there's the elevation of "punk" hair styles into "fun" hair with new shades of pink and orange. For the less brave, there are streaks and tipping, the more extreme of which can be seen on zebra-striped hair.

For those who've yet to reach puberty, there are the severed heads with "practice" hair colors to change the color of the hair.

Neither do the men escape. They are counseled "not to go gray." By not "being gray," they can avoid "looking old" and can "impress the boss" and thereby gain youth, admiration, and success. Commercials show a sallow, sullen man with dull gray hair that looks as though it was dusted with the day's floor-sweepings in lighting that casts shadows that would delight Boris Karloff's creepiest character.

Then, as the man combs stuff through his hair, his face and the lighting brighten. At the end of his daily combing, the man emerges renewed and smiling in makeup and lighting that wash away all the shadows. His new confidence glows like a halo. His wife is shown being kittenish and filled with admiration for this new man. His boss is so impressed he does a double-take, and you just know this no-longer-sullen or defeated man is in line for a promotion and a heck of a raise.

Although many of the graying men of the movies are still being dipped in the dye pots, a remarkable number of males of a certain age who have gained prominence on television have abandoned the dye pots and allowed their hair to go gray and even white—and look a lot better than the sullen model who apparently needed a lot of combing before he could be coaxed to smile.

Women, however, have been less fortunate in their role models. The brainwash of "gray is old" has taken hold so solidly that colored hair—any color but gray—has become a defense rather than a choice.

One attractive female model with an enviably maintained and bikini-worthy body, who broke new ground in introducing models of "a certain age" in roles other than those shown stricken with arthritis and constipation, was berated by a woman caller for allowing her hair to go gray.

Another woman wrote to Ann Landers saying she knew the columnist had "a very big birthday in July" and, having seen her on TV several times, felt that the reason Ms. Landers looked so youthful was that she had never allowed herself to go gray. The woman also wanted to know what Ms.

Landers used to keep her hair colored. Ms. Landers replied that her hairdresser, Brian Blanchard, told her it's Clairol-42.

Since the general perception of hair that has turned silver, no matter at what age, is associated with the *wrong* age for women in particular, those who feel they must conform, or who decide they like themselves better with a color other than their own, would be wise to become informed users of the products offered. It is not without reason that permanent hair dyes carry the most frightening label of all cosmetics.

The blinding of one woman in 1933 and the death of another from Lash Lure, an eyelash dye that used a synthetic aniline dye, such as the coal-tar dyes used in today's permanent hair dyes, led to the addition of cosmetics to the Food and Drug Law and the passage of the 1938 Food, Drug, and Cosmetic Act.

After five years of dragging atrocities through congressional hearings, Congress capitulated to the industry and exempted coal-tar hair dyes from the Act with the provision that the packages contain a cautionary statement—a statement not likely to be seen by the many who have their hair dyed in beauty salons and barbershops.

Since 1938, the Food, Drug, and Cosmetic Act has read:

A cosmetic shall be deemed to be adulterated—(a) If it bears or contains any poisonous or deleterious substance which may render it injurious to users under the conditions of use prescribed in the labeling thereof, or under such conditions of use as are customary or usual: *Provided,* that the provision shall not apply to coal-tar hair dye, the label of which bears the following legend conspicuously displayed thereon:

"Caution—This product contains ingredients which may cause skin irritation on certain individuals and a preliminary test according to accompanying directions should first be made. This product must not be used for dyeing the eyelashes or eyebrows; to do so may cause blindness," and the labeling of which bears

adequate directions for such preliminary testing. For the purposes of this paragraph . . . the term "hair dye" shall not include eyelash dyes or eyebrow dyes.

The "test" that provided the escape hatch for hair dyes is a patch test for allergy. This is done by washing a spot about the size of a quarter behind the ear or in the crook of the elbow, adding a drop of the dye mixture to be used, and leaving it intact without washing it off for twenty-four hours. If there is no redness, rash, swelling, or other reaction from the mixture, the manufacturers claim the hair dye can be used without risking an allergic reaction.

The test was intended as a check before *every* hair dyeing because an allergic reaction can occur even after several nonreaction applications. An allergic reaction to a hair dye can be disabling, and caution alone should insure a preliminary patch test before *each* application. In practice, most beauticians give a patch test to first-time dyers; hardly any give patch tests on subsequent touch-ups.

The same precaution should be taken with semipermanent dyes, which usually wear away gradually with a number of shampoos. They also bear the warning label, which is unseen when the application is made in beauty salons where the dyes sometimes masquerade as semipermanent "tints" or "rinses."

As an FDA spokesman explained the exemption:

When this provision was written into the cosmetic chapter of the law in 1938, coal-tar-containing hair dyes were recognized as substances that caused a significant number of individuals to become sensitized upon using the products. Upon repeated use, the sensitized person develops an allergic reaction which may manifest itself in mild skin irritation in the area of the scalp or in many cases manifests itself as violent irritation accompanied by rash, fever, pustules in the scalp area which may become infected. The person who suffers a severe reaction is seriously ill and may require hospitalization followed by medical treatment for months.

However, the Congress concluded in 1938 that the patch test would enable individuals who became sensitized to the coal-tar hair dyes to safeguard themselves against that type of injury, and it decided that the widespread desire for a permanent-type hair dye was great enough to warrant the exemption provision which made it unnecessary for coal-tar hair dyes to be free from deleterious or poisonous substances.

Both the FDA and the hair dye industry now know that allergy is not the only "type of injury" that can result from the admitted poisonous and deleterious hair dyes.

One woman, who showed no adverse reaction to an initial patch test, dyed her hair about twenty times before she and her doctor realized something was wrong. Her illness was diagnosed as *periarteritis nodosa,* a serious disease involving the inflammation of tissue around the arteries. Patch tests had not been made before retouching, but it was pointed out that patch tests might only have shown a skin sensitivity to the dye—not the toxic systemic reaction the woman suffered. Consequently, the Missouri courts awarded damages to the injured woman in a decision against Roux Distributing Company.

Another woman claimed she became permanently bald as the result of a single application of Helena Rubinstein's Tintillate, a permanent-color shampoo tint. She also claimed she had followed instructions and had given herself a patch test that indicated no adverse reaction. The following day, she applied the dye to blend in some gray strands with her naturally red hair.

According to the thirty-three-year-old housewife, she noticed that her hair felt gummy as she set it in curlers. Three days later, a rash appeared around her neck, ears, and forehead. As she brushed her hair, she noticed that more and more of it caught in the bristles of the brush.

Within three months, the attactive mother of six lost all her hair, her eyebrows, and her eyelashes. Side effects also were alleged to have necessitated the removal of her right kidney six months after she had dyed her hair.

The Colorado woman filed a suit in Denver for $600,000 against Helena Rubinstein, Inc. et al, at which time attorney Robert Leland Johnson, co-counsel with Melvin M. Belli, noted that many women who had lost their hair using hair dye preparations were too embarrassed and emotionally upset to sue and to expose themselves to publicity.

Two years later, the suit was settled out of court for $23,500. The housewife said she's forced to wear a wig, paint on her eyebrows, and wear false eyelashes to simulate her former appearance.

Actress Carol Channing, whose allergies have so restricted her choice of food that she must carry her food with her, attributes her allergy problems to bleaches and hair coloring that caused her to lose her hair and to resort to wigs.

In 1978, the House of Representatives held hearings on cancer-causing chemicals and zeroed in on hair dyes. Laboratory tests, conducted by Dr. Bruce N. Ames and his associates in the biochemistry department of the University of California at Berkley, had shown a number of hair dye ingredients to be carcinogenic and mutagenic.

Even before retiring Congressman John E. Moss of California opened the hearings, the safety of some hair dye ingredients was being questioned. As early as 1955, reports had come from Japan of tests that showed 2,4-toluenediamine, a hair dye component also known as 2,4-TDA, caused cancerous growths to form at the point of contact when injected under the skin of rats.

In May 1969, *Cancer Research*, a Japanese scientific

journal, published the results of tests in which rats fed a 0.1 percent concentration of 2,4-TDA in food all developed liver cancers.

On September 14, 1970, *The National Observer* published an article headlined: "Cancer Suspect Is Confirmed in Many Hair Dyes." In it, August Gribbin reported the Japanese findings and added that tests conducted by Dr. Elizabeth Weisburger at the National Cancer Institute confirmed that 2,4-TDA injected under the skin of laboratory animals produced tumors.

Mr. Gribbin also reported: "Inquiries at the Food and Drug Adminstration, the agency most concerned with the safety of cosmetic products, turned up only official confusion. Nobody there seems to be aware of the findings at the Cancer Institute.

"But indications of 2,4-TDA's cancer-producing capability aren't new. The FDA has reports dating from 1949 that not only 2,4-TDA but several other toluenediamine compounds . . . can produce cancer in animals."

As a fixative used mostly in the dark shades of permanent and semipermanent hair dyes, 2,4-TDA had substitutes or alternates that could be used without appreciably changing the efficacy of the hair dyes.

According to Mr. Gribbin: "It need not be included at all. But officials of [several large companies selling hair dyes] say 2,4-TDA is routinely used in many of the 43 brands of permanent or semipermanent hair dyes marketed by the nation's 32 hair-dye manufacturers."

He added that, although most of the estimated 70 million Americans who were coloring their hair were using rinses, about eight million were using dyes that might contain 2,4-TDA, and those dyes "can easily get under the skin through scalp cuts or sores."

Two weeks after the article appeared, a joint meeting of

FDA and cosmetic industry representatives resulted in the FDA beginning an 18-month testing program to determine the effects of 2,4-TDA when painted on the skin of mice, and its penetrability, if any, through human skin.

Dr. Francis N. Marzulli, FDA chief dermatoxicologist in charge of the tests, hoped to find out more about the effects of the fixative in addition to its carcinogenic dangers. He sought to find out why, when a rash appeared on the user of a hair dye as an allergic reaction, it sometimes appeared not only at the site of application, but also under the breasts, in the pubic areas, and on other parts of the body.

The tests sought also to explain why women using two kinds of dyes from a leading hair dye manufacturer complained of passing black urine. Some men who dyed their hair also found their urine turning black.

Although the FDA reported that painting the skin of mice with the dyes also turned the mice's urine black, neither the agency nor the manufacturer was able to find an explanation.

Mr. Gribbin quoted Dr. Marzulli as saying it was "a ten-year analytic problem." He also quoted the hair dye company as claiming to have spent $500,000 in testing. Finding no explanation, they continued the product without alteration.

In 1977, twenty-two years after the Japanese studies found 2,4-TDA to be carcinogenic—and twenty-eight years from FDA's reported knowledge—the General Accounting Office said, "Most cosmetic manufacturers stopped using toluene-2,4-diamine [2,4-TDA] in hair dyes after it was found to cause cancer in laboratory animals. However, data submitted to FDA under its voluntary program for filing cosmetic product ingredient statements indicates that it is still used in at least seven permanent hair dyes."

An FDA proposal to ban the use of 2,4-TDA in hair dyes later floundered and sputtered in the *Federal Register* without a final resolution. Meanwhile, packages containing dyes with the disgraced ingredient were not recalled and remained on the shelves to be carried away by unsuspecting consumers.

In 1975, Dr. Bruce Ames found 2,4-TDA to be mutagenic as well as carcinogenic. The now famous and accepted Ames Test uses bacteria such as salmonella to determine genetic changes.

The Ames hair dye discoveries that shook industry and government agencies alike resulted from what began as a routine biochemistry class experiment at the University of California. Hundreds of commercial products were tested for mutagenicity. According to Dr. Ames, "Only two products were found to be mutagenic: cigarette smoke tar and an oxidative-type [permanent] hair dye."

Interviewed prior to the Moss Hearings, Dr. Ames was asked if he believed a substance that was "simply a mutagen" would be harmful to persons exposed to it.

Dr. Ames said he believed it would be harmful. "Even if they weren't carcinogens, mutagens are substances that damage the genes, and if they get to the human germ line then they would cause birth defects in our children and grandchildren. Already 5 to 10 percent of births have some kind of genetic abnormality. Mutagenesis is a serious problem even distinct from carcinogenesis, but there seems to be a tremendous overlap between chemicals that are mutagens and carcinogens. In fact, the favored theory on why this is, is that most chemicals that cause cancer are actually carcinogenic because they are mutagens, because they damage the DNA of our somatic cells. A cell with a particular damage to its DNA could have a control mechanism damaged so that the cell keeps on growing when it's not supposed to and gives rise to a tumor."

Concentrating on the most used permanent dyes, Dr. Ames' students tested about thirty formulations from the lines of eight companies: Alberto-Culver Co. (For Brunettes Only); John H. Breck, Inc.; Clairol Inc.; Cosmair, Inc. (L'Oreal); The Gillette Co. (Toni); Revlon; Roux Laboratories, Inc.; and Tussy Cosmetics, Inc. (Ogilvie). Mutagenic hair dyes were reportedly found in every hair dye product line tested.

Out of eighteen chemicals used in the United States in oxidative, or permanent, hair dyes, nine were found to be mutagenic: 2,4-diaminoanisole, 4-nitro-o-phenylenediamine, 2-nitro-p-phenylenediamine, 2,5-diaminoanisole, 2-amino- 5-nitrophenol, m-phenylenediamine, o-phenylenediamine, 2-amino-4-nitrophenol, and 2,5-diaminotoluene. These were in addition to 2,4-TDA, which Dr. Ames had been told was no longer being used.

The tests further showed that 150 out of 169 permanent hair dyes tested were mutagenic. Topping the list as the most potent mutagen of the mutagenic components was 2,4-diaminoanisole (2,4-DAA), also known as 4-methoxy-m-phenylenediamine (4-MMPD), which Dr. Ames said was a close relative of 2,4-TDA—*and thirty times more active!* The Environmental Defense Fund, the independent consumer group, found there were more than 400 hair dyes with 2,4-DAA currently on the market.

Dr. Ames found 2,4-DAA "particularly interesting because it has practically the same structure as [2,4-TDA] . . . On the surface it seems as if an untested chemical (2,4-DAA) that's very close in structure to one that was shown to be a carcinogen [2,4-TDA] was used as a replacement.

"I don't know whether that's true or not, but there's certainly a lot of it in hair dyes, and it performs the same function in hair dyes, as far as I understand, as the 2,4-diaminotoluene. Anyway, it was quite a good mutagen in our system, even better than the [2,4-TDA]. 2,4-diaminoanisole is now coming out as a carcinogen in animals just the way 2,4-diaminotoluene did."

Industry representatives confirmed the fact that there was "a lot" of 2,4-DAA in hair dyes.

During the 1978 congressional hearings, Dr. John F. Corbett, chairman of CTFA's Hair Dye Technical Committee and Clairol's Technical Development vice-president, estimated that 15,000 pounds of 2,4-DAA were used in hair dyes, compared to 100 pounds of 2,4-TDA, in a year.

In an exchange with Congressman Andrew Maguire in which the congressman sought to establish why the industry had removed 2,4-TDA when it became suspect and apparently intended to do nothing about the now suspect 2,4-DAA, Dr. Corbett admitted: "In 1970, we had no data on 2,4-TDA. We did not even bother to gather data on 2,4-TDA, but we removed it from our product there and then.

"I would not be prepared to fall back on the epidemiological evidence of a long-term exposure of the whole female hair dye user population to 100 pounds a year, but I am certainly prepared to fall back on it in respect of such widespread uses as has occurred with 2,4-diaminoanisole."

Congressman Maguire turned to the then CTFA president, James H. Merritt, who had accompanied Dr. Corbett to the witness table along with CTFA Science Vice-President Norman H. Estrin and CTFA Counsel Peter Barton Hutt, who had alternated from industry to FDA and back to representing industry in a few short years.

Maguire: Mr. Merritt, do you have an answer to the question?

Merritt: I think you have to look at the benefit and balance it with the risk involved.

Maguire: How do you justify the difference between TDA and

DAA, Mr. Merritt? One has been taken out and the other has been left in.

Merritt: At the time TDA was removed, it was because there was an alternative. But with respect to the other, there is no alternative.

Maguire: There is no alternative?

Merritt: That is correct.

Maguire: Have you pursued, over the last 40 years, since you received your exemption for hair dyes, a study of alternatives?

Merritt: I am sure the industry has looked at every possible chemical for use in hair dyes.

Minutes before, Dr. Corbett had testified that he "could make a hair dye today that does not use 2,4-diaminoanisole."

Sure enough, after 2,4-DAA made headlines, Clairol, the company employing Dr. Corbett, came out with hair dyes that did not have 2,4-DAA, but not before Cosmair beat it to the market with L'Oreal hair dyes minus the challenged ingredient. The old hair dyes with 2,4-DAA, however, remained in the market—lots of them, for a long time—to be bought and used by the unwary, uninformed, or careless buyer.

At the local hairdresser, even the best informed would-be dyer could not tell which dye was the old or new formula. Neither could the local hairdresser. The professional-use packages were exempt from ingredient labeling, and neither Cosmair nor Clairol had voluntarily labeled the ingredients for the local hairdresser.

In eliminating 2,4-DAA, Clairol and Cosmair claimed they had done so to avoid having the dyes subjected to a possible warning label, and not because they believed the ingredient was dangerous.

The warning label was originally proposed by the Environmental Defense Fund in a citizen petition to the FDA, citing National Cancer Institute experiments as reason to require a cancer warning. The NCI tests indicated "that 2,4-DAA causes a statistically significant increase in site-specific tumors in male and female rats and mice, and must therefore be considered carcinogenic in both mammalian species."

The October 17, 1977 petition requested the FDA commissioner to "immediately promulgate a rule ... requiring the following warning:

> This product contains the chemical 2,4-DAA, which can enter your bloodstream through your scalp and has been shown to cause cancer in animals."

On January 6, 1978, the FDA published its own proposal to require hair dyes with 2,4-DAA to carry the label warning:

> Contains an ingredient that can penetrate your skin and has been determined to cause cancer in laboratory animals.

The FDA also proposed a poster warning to be posted in beauty shops to read:

> Some hair dyes contain ingredients which may cause cancer. These hair dyes are required to bear a label warning. Ask to see the label of the product intended for your hair.

Two days before the FDA proposal appeared in the *Federal Register*, the CTFA began its objections for the industry. And, again, an FDA proposal joined the mothball army of FDA proposals, destined never to attain the rank of active regulation.

In the factories, in the stores, and in the beauty shops it was business as usual. After all, there was nothing to stop hair dye companies from *legally* incorporating carcinogens, mutagens, or anything else in their products.

Congress itself had exempted them from any legal responsibility when it exempted coal-tar hair dyes from complying with any of the meager rules of the cosmetic game. That Congress did not go beyond allergic reactions was to the industry's advantage and the consumer's disadvantage. The hair dye industry had won the game, and it did not intend to give up any of its winnings.

The National Cancer Institute (NCI) had more than 2,4-DAA and 2,4-TDA on its cancer-suspect list. Out of thirteen hair dye ingredients in the NCI bioassays, the preliminary results indicated six were carcinogens.

Direct black and direct blue, two of several benzidine-derived dyes used in some temporary and semipermanent hair dyes, caught the CTFA in an unintended or intended deception—a charge characteristically used by the CTFA against others to deflect any criticism of the industry it represents. When the two colors appeared on the NCI cancer list, CTFA rushed to tell reporters that no major manufacturer had used the benzidine-derived colors in hair dyes since 1973.

CTFA was promptly proved wrong when personnel from the General Accounting Office bought eight temporary hair dyes containing one or more benzidine-derived colors at the local drugstores. All were from Roux Laboratories, a major producer of hair dyes and a CTFA member.

An NCI interim report on the two colors noted that ninety-day tests on animals found:

> In the short-term feeding studies, [the two] dyes produced liver toxicity in both species. Cancerous and precancerous conditions were found in rats, similar to the damage produced by known liver carcinogens.

> In addition, though the dyes were benzidine free when fed to the animals, benzidine was found in the urine of dosed rats

and mice, and indication that animal systems break down the dyes and release benzidine.

Because the effects were so striking in the brief trial period and in comparatively young animals, NCI scientists resolved that findings should be reported, in order to expedite investigation of human exposures and the possible risks involved.

Benzidine, from which the colors were derived, is defined in *The Merck Index*: "White or slightly reddish [crystalline] powder; darkens on exposure to air and light. *Poisonous!*—Solid and vapor are rapidly absorbed through skin.—Human Toxicity: May cause injury to blood and is suspected as a cause of bladder tumors. On ingestion may produce nausea and vomiting, liver and kidney damage."

The subject of the benzidine-derived dyes and why they remained on the market when the public had been misled into believing they'd been discontinued erupted into a heated debate between Congressman Henry A. Waxman and Dr. Corbett, with interspersed remarks from Chairman Moss and CTFA President Merritt.

The Corbett-Merritt team tried its well-rehearsed deflective gambit, but the Waxman-Moss team would not be deflected.

After a lengthy, finger-pointing speech in which Dr. Corbett tried to deflect the questioning on the carcinogenic dyes to cancer-promoting cigarettes, diet, radiation, and ultraviolet light—a ploy used by cosmetic industry spokesmen for at least the twenty-five years I've been listening to them—Congressman Waxman brought him sharply back to the subject.

Waxman: You obviously can "out-science" talk me. But this is a product [indicating] that one of my aides purchased off the shelf in a retail establishment here in Washington, D.C.

It contains a chemical called "Direct Blue 6" which was the subject of the recent NCI study. NCI found it to be highly carcinogenic. They determined that here was a danger because "Direct Blue 6" may be absorbed through the skin.

You told me that the industry is no longer manufacturing products containing this chemical. Is that correct?

Corbett: That is what I understand, yes.

Waxman: Why don't you know why the industry has stopped manufacturing hair dye products containing "Direct Blue 6"? Why can't you tell us whether it is due to a recognition of the potential health danger which you refuse to acknowledge?

Merritt: I might interject, please.

Moss: Let us wait for the response.

Waxman: This is a scientist from the cosmetic industry and I want to find out why some of the members of the industry do not know what others are doing and why they have not voluntarily taken benzidine-derived dyes off the market.

Corbett: That is commercial information. I will try to find out. I think it may be just prudent business sense that made them take if off.

Waxman: I think it is prudent business sense not to put something on the market that contains benzidine—a substance we know is clearly carcinogenic. I think we found out that this is a serious enough matter that tumors were found in test animals after only 90 days. NCI concluded these dyes were potent carcinogens and may well be dangerous.

Then you tell me you do not even know why the industry took the dyes off the market. This bottle of hair dye rinse [Roux Fanci-full Rinse] was purchased within the last couple of days. People right now are able to purchase products containing benzidine.

Corbett: With due respect, I am under oath and I do not know the reason they took it off. I have not discussed it with them.

Waxman: Are you aware of the fact that Japan banned benzidine in 1971?

Corbett: But this does not contain benzidine. It contains diaso dyes that are derived from benzidine. They, in chemical character, are different from benzidine itself.

Waxman: They are derivatives, are they not?

Corbett: Yes, but that is the same as saying aspirin is a benzidine derivative. It does not mean anything.

Waxman: Did not NCI determine that benzidine-based dyes convert to benzidine in the human body?

Corbett: When ingested, yes.

Waxman: The question, then, is whether it is ingested.

Corbett: I said that.

Waxman: Mr. Merritt, your testimony is: To the vast majority of consumers, the contributions of cosmetics to self-assurance and self-esteem are as important as the nutritional and medical benefits of food and drugs.

Are you telling us that it is as important, that is, that it is more important to look good than to feel good?

Merritt: I think looking good and feeling good perhaps could be equally important to many people. On the other hand, there are certain individuals to which one might be better than the other.

Waxman: Really? I see. So, some individuals ought to have cancer and others not?

Merritt: You are taking that out of context.

Waxman: I am disturbed by your willingness to make the evaluation that for some people it is so important to look good that it is worth taking the risk that they are going to get cancer. I find that appalling. Is that what you are saying?

Merritt: No, not in that context. What about cigarettes?

Waxman: Aren't you just throwing some smoke up in the air?

Moss: With all due respect, we are not dealing with cigarettes today. We have wrestled with that problem over a period of time in the past. We will do it again, but not today.

At the close of the hearings, Drs. Ames and Corbett and a few others were interviewed on radio and television.

Dr. Ames told viewers and listeners there was evidence that some hair dyes might not only cause cancer and damage to future generations, if one were to take the nonhuman tests as warning to human beings; they might also cause birth defects in the immediate generation. He advised women who might be pregnant to refrain from dyeing their hair while they were pregnant in deference to the children to come.

Dr. Corbett repeated his well-rehearsed dissertations on the safety of hair dyes and cosmetics and how a person would have to drink gallons of the stuff before one need worry about consequences. He neglected to explain that, whether a substance is drunk or absorbed through the skin, the results are the same—the substance is in the bloodstream—and that many cosmetic chemicals had been found to have been absorbed through human skin. Then, too, there was that black urine for days after the hair-dyeing—acknowledged by the manufacturer and the FDA. Surely those men and women had not drunk the dye.

Leslie Dach, EDF science associate, and others reminded all concerned that cancer is not an immediate visible reaction that can be detected the way a rash or a pimple can. It may be twenty years or longer before cancer makes itself known—long enough for the cosmetic industry to deny responsibility.

A number of bills asking for the elimination of the hair dye exemption were thrown into the hopper—and died there.

The question remains: How much help is the public getting from its legislators and regulators in keeping potentially dangerous products out of the market and off the store shelves? And how much help can we expect in sorting the reasonably safe from the questionably unsafe?

Take, for instance, the so-called "color restorers" that use lead acetate to coat the hair in much the same way rust forms on metal. Harry Raybin, former director of the New York City Poison Control Center, said the lead-containing "color restorer" liquids and pomades should not be allowed on the market.

The lead-based preparations are combed into the hair, leaving a residue on both hair and comb. Since, as Mr. Raybin pointed out, infants and children often play with combs, the residue is apt to end up in the infants and children. Accidental swallowing of creams or liquids containing substantial amounts of lead increases the potential hazard of stultifying damage to a child's brain.

Some of the "color restorers," which until 1977 did not have to list or disclose ingredients, were found to contain 10 to 25 percent lead acetate.

The Federal Trade Commission could make a case for misleading advertising, since the products do not "restore" color but merely coat hair with lead salt, making the hair progressively darker. In no way does it *restore* the previous hair color.

The FDA might also prove the products to be mislabeled on the same premise. Instead, in 1981, the FDA approved the permanent listing of lead-acetate used in the "restorers" as a color additive and announced that it could even bypass the certification required of other color additives. The puzzling action came after lead acetate had been on the provisional color additives list since 1960, when the passage of the Color Additives Amendment required new testing to prove safety.

By the FDA's own account, "FDA issued a notice in response to industry petitions in which metallic salt and vegetable color manufacturers were advised that their products were not eligible for the coal-tar dye exemption to the premarket clearance requirements of the Amendments and that these colorants were color additives subject to all the requirements of the Amendments."

FDA also asked for data so that a determination could be made whether the additives could be permanently listed for use. In the meantime, the agency promised not to take any regulatory action against the additives and the companies could go on using them.

Only the vegetable-base henna responded with a petition for listing, which it was given.

Ten year later, the FDA posted a reminder notice in the *Federal Register*. In January 1973, it said that only those metallic salts or vegetable colorants for which petitions had been filed by July 30, 1973, could continue to be marketed. This prompted the Committee of the Progressive Hair Dye Industry to petition for listing.

FDA put lead acetate on the provisional list and then postponed permanent listing while the "color restorers" went on testing. Through animal feedings in the 1950s and 1960s, it had been established "conclusively" that lead acetate was carcinogenic in mice and rats. However, the FDA claimed that, since human epidemiological data was limited and considered equivocal, "a conclusion whether lead was a human carcinogen could not be reached."

As things were, the Delaney Amendment prevented the legal use of any color additive, ingested or absorbed through the skin, that was shown to be a carcinogen to man or animal. As matters developed in the 1980s, the FDA joined the progressive-dye industry (which chose to call its products "color restorers" instead of "progressive dyes") in circumventing the Delaney Amendment, which had the bad taste to favor consumers.

Yes, said the FDA, *lead acetate was definitely an animal carcinogen and it might be a human carcinogen. Yes,* said the FDA, *it was absorbed through the scalp.* But by 1981, the new policy shattered the Delaney Amendment without even a vote from Congress. The one-in-a-million risk was in. And, anyway, according to industry tests, only a little bit of lead was absorbed through the scalp.

Then a very curious thing happened in explaining the FDA's new stance. The arguments the FDA used were arguments the CTFA and the cosmetic industry had used for decades—the same hoary "look at the other guys" rationalizations that had been flattened in the War on Cancer Hearings.

Apparently, in 1981, it no longer mattered that consumers got a little more lead into their bodies. After all, they were already getting a dose of lead from food, water, and air.

Some consumer objections were filed and were dismissed by the FDA. Barely mentioned was the fact that arsenic and mercury were also a part of the "color restorer" formulas.

Both arsenic and mercury are known to be toxic and dangerous to the human system; and a while back, Switzerland banned lead and mercury in cosmetics. In 1981, however, the U.S. "consumer protective" agency not only gave manufacturers permission to use arsenic and mercury along with the carcinogenic lead acetate, it freed the color additive from the certification legally required of other color additives. Consequently, although the FDA set guidelines for quantities to be used in the progressive dyes, without its certifying the batches the public has no assurance that these guidelines are being met.

In 1979, Heinz Eiermann, FDA's director of Cosmetics Technology, flew to Chile to tell a Latin-American convention of cosmetic chemists: "The risk of cancer is determined by the cancer incidence in a bioassay and the degree of exposure; and it is believed that no threshold exists below which cancer is not expected to occur. Accordingly, even a minute amount of a carcinogen, possibly present in a cosmetic as a contaminant, may be expected to cause cancer in the exposed population, though the number of cases may be extremely small."

In 1980 and 1981, the FDA was singing industry's song, eager to explain how few consumers would be sacrificed to a free and easy "color restorer." Mouthing industry's words of how little lead would leak into the brain and bloodstream through an intact scalp, the decision makers apparently ignored the fact that lead salts continuously combed through the hair are apt to cause the scalp to itch and the person beneath the scalp to scratch. It might, in fact, be difficult to find many intact scalps among the progressive dye habitués. And despite warning labels, how many would remember to wash their hands and clean off their skin after every combing—or to hide the combs and brushes so that the nonuser children would be protected from adding just a little more lead than they might otherwise get from the duly blamed food, water, and air?

QUESTIONS AND ANSWERS

I'm a hairdresser in a beauty shop, and some of my customers ask me about ingredients they've read about and want to know if those ingredients are in the products I'm using. I have to tell them that I don't know because the ingredients aren't listed on most the packages we buy. How can I find out what the ingredients are in our supplies so that I will have that information for our customers?

Since professional packages are exempted from ingredient labeling, I suggest you write to the manufacturer or distributor for a list of ingredients used. The ingredients should be readily available since most of your supplies are duplicated in retail products sold over the counter to the general public. If they are not, write to the Cosmetic Division of the Food and Drug Administration in Washington, D.C.

I've decided that I want to color my hair. Since this is the first time I'll be coloring my hair, how do you suggest I go about it?

First, take yourself to the wig department of a department store—preferably the kind where they leave you alone—

to try on various wigs in shades of color you're considering for your hair. Take your time to decide what and if you really like another color with your skin coloring. If you find a bargain-basement wig for a few dollars in a color you think is right, you might consider buying it and wearing it around the house to see if the color really is right for you. You might also get a consensus of opinions on it from people you trust and who are close to you.

Once you decide on a color and a shade of that color, try a temporary rinse first. If you hate it, you can wash it out. It won't be that easy with a permanent hair color.

I'd then try a semipermanent hair color—the kind that washes out in a number of shampoos. You might want to do this with a professional hairdresser. Whatever you decide, be sure you have a patch test with the mixture to be used, twenty-four hours before the actual application.

After you've lived with the color through the shampoos, you should have a pretty good idea whether you want to make the change. You may find that you can continue with the semipermanent dye, which is a lot easier to live with since it eliminates the definite demarcation between the roots and the artificial color.

If you feel you must go on to a permanent dye, I suggest you have at least your first few applications done professionally. Again, just be sure you have a patch test before each application.

I prefer to dye my own hair. Have you any suggestions about application?

Treat every application of hair dye of any kind defensively. Follow instructions for giving yourself a patch test before every application and try a strand test to see if the color is right. If there is any irritation, burning, redness, rash, or swelling from the patch test, don't go ahead with the hair dye.

Usually, there's an 800 telephone number for consumer questions given in the package insert. If the dye isn't right for you, you'll probably be told to return the package to the store or the manufacturer for another product or a refund.

Once you're safely past the patch and strand tests, go ahead with the application carefully, following instructions. However, although most hair dye instructions tell you to pour the liquid on your hair as you section it, I suggest that you pour the mixture into a nonmetal bowl and use a natural-bristle brush (an old toothbrush will do) to take up and apply the color. There is no need to pour the dye on your scalp. You're trying to color your hair, not your scalp.

Keep your eyes tightly shut while you're rinsing the dye out of your hair. Then shampoo thoroughly.

I find that when I color my own hair, which is fairly short, I don't need a whole bottle for an application. Yet the instructions tell you to throw out the mixture because it might explode if you try to save it.

As long as you don't mix the hair color and the developer, you can recap the two bottles and keep them. Next time, try mixing just half of each. You can always go back and mix more if you need more. Whatever you mix must be used or discarded.

I'm not happy with the shade I'm using. Can I mix two shades of a color?

Yes. Mix only the color if you want to recap and save the extra. Then, mix the right amount with the developer.

How can I tone down the red in a color?

Add a drabber to the color mixture, according to directions. Drabbers are made for light and dark shades. Get the one that is appropriate to the color you're using.

What can I do if I find that I don't like the color after I've applied it?

If you want to make the color darker, you can redye your hair with a darker dye. If the color is darker than you want it, you cannot dye it lighter. You must strip the color and then recolor it. However, this will not restore your hair to its former color, which will have been stripped to a lemon yellow or a variation. I strongly recommend against this unless it's absolutely necessary—then, if it is, to have it done professionally.

What is a two-process coloring?

This is a process that's used in changing dark hair into light or blond. The dark color is first removed and then the desired shade is applied, usually in the form of a toner. This is a process that is better left to professionals.

How do I choose the right shampoo for my hair?

Most shampoos are labeled for "dry," "normal," "oily," or "color-treated" hair. Then there are the "special" ingredients, ranging from the jojoba bean to placenta, which is the residue from somebody's or some animal's afterbirth.

Just remember that the speck or dollop of "special" ingredient is washed in and out. Most are there to tempt you into believing more than they can deliver. The basic shampoo is the one that does the job.

Buy the smallest size of the least expensive shampoo in your hair's category. If it works well, buy the larger size and continue using it. There's no need to wash a lot of dollars down the drain.

We live in an area that has rather hard water. Even with a water softener, I find it difficult to get all the soap or shampoo rinsed out of my hair.

After your preliminary rinsing, try a rinse of approximately one part white vinegar to four parts water, then rinse again. Keep your eyes tightly shut during the vinegar rinse. Vinegar stings if it gets in your eyes. If you prefer it, lemon juice can be used instead of vinegar.

I am confused with so many hair treatments and conditioners on the market. Since I've been dyeing my hair, I find that my hair becomes matted during my shampooing and that it is quite dry. I think my hair can use some help.

Why not try something you probably have in your refrigerator? After shampooing, and without trying to comb your matted hair, work some mayonnaise into the strands. Then cover your hair with a plastic wrap, cap, or bag. Wait about ten minutes, or longer if you think you need it.

Rinse well with warm water, using a vinegar rinse for your next-to-last rinse, and you'll find you can comb your hair without snarls so that you can go on with your usual setting or styling.

If you've been overly generous with the mayonnaise, you may have to give your hair a light shampoo before the rinsing. Also, try to avoid blow dryers or any other dryers, as well as teasing.

17

The Skin

No other part of the body is so mistreated
as the skin.
—Dr. Veronica L. Conley,
Former Assistant Secretary,
Committee on Cosmetics,
American Medical Association

Hope is what we sell in cosmetics.
—Stephen L. Mayham,
Past Honorary President,
The Toilet Goods Association

Many women's dressers [are] cluttered with
"dead enthusiasm"—stale jars, unopened bottles,
half-used boxes of cosmetics.
—Vance Packard,
The Hidden Persuaders

As "going gray" has become a dreaded condition, so, too, has "aging" become a visitation worse than death. In a macabre dance, the cosmetic industry dangles the threat of "aging" over the heads of born-beautiful young models, and holds out hope for evading the monster with a jar of "priceless" cream, precisely priced.

In a commercial, with what probably was thought to be a daring approach, one company hired French actress Catherine Deneuve, who previously had been Chanel No. 5's enticer, to tell the television cameras to "come closer." As the camera "came closer," she explained that she was used to being looked at, and boasted that a new cream was going to keep her looking the way she did even while she confessed to being forty. Off camera, Ms. Deneuve is reported to have said how much she feared getting old.

Despite the many "scientific breakthroughs" regularly announced by cosmetic companies for a multitude of "new discovery" products, people still stubbornly grow older instead of younger. Yet the cosmetic industry has been eminently successful in holding out the carrot of youth a lucrative nose-length away with the promise that youth can be had for the price of its newest discovery, born of science, rediscovered from the ancient hills or the Dead Sea, wrested from exotic herbs, or brought forth from the tombs of Cleopatra or Nefertiti, both of whom apparently died before they got old and, thereby, effectively escaped looking old while they lived.

Skin, the more or less twenty square feet of it that holds each of us together in nature's unique and unparalleled packaging, is the cosmetic industry's prime target for selling hope along with its products. In the past decade, "treatment" products have raced ahead of perfumes in creating the widest profit margins between product and price.

There are "treatments" now for skin in infancy when it manifests its peevishness in diaper rash and chafing, through the heartaches of its acting up in adolescence; and then, without waiting a decent interval, the cosmetic industry throws females immediately into the age of anxiety.

"IT'S NEVER TOO SOON TO START," Charles of the Ritz admonishes. "Why wait? You may not even be aware of it now, it's so subtle. Those tiny, tiny lines. Barely noticeable today ..." The windup claims "every woman needs Age-Zone Controller."

Lancôme brings Frenchship with *Progrès Plus Creme*

Anti-Rides, its ambiguous "proven challenge to wrinkles" that promises to help the skin to help itself in preventing "dehydrating signs of aging." Lancôme's promise is illustrated by Isabella Rossellini, the exquisite young daughter of Ingrid Bergman and Roberto Rossellini, who obviously has experienced no "dehydrating signs of aging" and owes her unwrinkled beauty to her age and extraordinary genes.

Stendhal, with more Frenchship, counsels, "The sea can help you slow the ravages of time," and changes the message to sell two creams, one for day and one for night. In addition to corralling "natural marine extracts," Stendhal throws in "hop, horse-tail and horse chestnut," indicating the sea was at a very high tide.

Not to be outdone, Estée Lauder "bring you Age-Controlling Creme" with the same model she's used for some years but who now looks different than she did her first time out.

Yet, for all the proclaimed new "breakthroughs," the words have a familiar ring. They are the same as those that prompted me to begin asking simple questions about the heralded "proof" and "clinical tests," and about the "scientific miracles" of the 1960s. Only the names and the prices have changed.

Where are yesterday's breakthrough creams, cremes, and potions that were to make us younger and better—or, at least, keep us the same today as we were yesterday? Where are the dollars we spent on yesterday's promises?

A few years ago, the claims being made for the current crop of cosmetic "treatment" products would have alerted the FDA to declare the "treatments" to be drugs and subject to the stricter drug regulations, and the FTC to ask for proof of those claims. However, the "treatment" purveyors apparently are confident enough that their political action committee has created friends in high places and of the pressure on the agencies to follow the administration-dictated, closed-eye policy to sail their claims farther and farther into the unchartered seas of hope and dollars.

Today's "treatments" are replete with claims of effecting the normal function or structure of the body—claims that normally would effect the normal actions of an alert FTC and FDA. The more cautious "treatment" purveyors also know enough to put their probable drug claims in their advertising, where the FTC is nominally in charge but has been comatose for the past decade, and to keep the claims off the labeling, which even now may twitch the FDA into action.

Among the claims being made are those of Charles of the Ritz, whose Age-Zone Controller "Diminishes lines, accelerates cell renewal as it penetrates deeply." Lancôme Progrès Plus Creme Anti-Rides (part of Cosmair of the L'Oreal hair dye, etc. complex) has a "me-too" claim in "The proven capacity to diminish wrinkles by reducing their length and depth" and "The acceleration of your skin's natural cell renewal activities." It also adds "A barrier against collagen breakdown to deter the formation of wrinkles."

Again, not to be outdone by others' claims, Estée Lauder pitches Age-Controlling Creme, claiming it contains "Sodium RNA, an active ingredient that helps speed up the skin's natural cell renewal process to a rate that existed when your skin was younger" and adds a "patented natural protein complex" that "interacts with your skin's own natural protein . . ."

French Orlane claims its Estrait Vital "goes beyond repair"; it "Helps speed fresh cells to the surface" and "Helps restructure the skin to a new fullness and smoothness."

Heady-sounding claims. Back from the late 1950s and the 1960s are the "clinical tests," the "distinguished laboratories," the inference of "medical" help without an office visit. Irma Shorell, daughter of a plastic surgeon, presses that her creams are "based on the research of a world famous Plastic Surgeon." Coty claims its Overnight Cellular Replacement Cream is "So effective—improvement begins overnight. Yet you don't need a doctor's prescription."

To the casual reader, it may sound as though there have been really important scientific and medical discoveries. To those who have been industry watchers for the past quarter-century, the claims evoke a feeling of déjà vu.

Actually, the most important and acknowledged semi-discovery has been the confirmation that surface ingredients, other than drugs, can penetrate an intact skin. How beneficial or hazardous the uncontrolled absorption of a chemical may be depends on what is being absorbed, whether such absorption creates systemic changes, and, if so, what happens or may be expected to happen in time.

Since Dr. Joseph Faucher of Union Carbide Corporation told a gathering of cosmetic chemists in 1978 that his tests showed that "a fair amount" of shampoo went into the scalp after it had been left on for one minute, there have been a number of seminars and symposiums on skin penetration. There also has been general confirmation and general bewilderment beyond advertising simplistics. Obviously, in order to find out what happens with the absorption of countless ingredients and countless combinations of ingredients, testing is needed—testing that now is not required of any product classified as a cosmetic.

Although many, if not most, of the larger, well-known companies do some testing, the question remains how and how much they test and how much they know about the beneficial and, perhaps, deleterious effects of absorption. Despite the many papers being read and published on the new theory of skin and scalp penetration, little has surfaced beyond theory and methods of testing. There are no announcements of long-term studies that might determine what, if any, would be the effects of "negligible" one-in-a-million risk-assessed ingredients.

One food and drug human clinic laboratory regularly advertises for men and women of all ages. One wonders how many would volunteer to test products if they were told there was a one-in-a-million chance that they might get cancer from an ingredient. After all, there are daily lotteries where the chances of winning are much less than one in a million, yet someone wins the prize.

Without required testing of ingredients and products before they are marketed, there is an abysmal lack of knowledge even on the part of the manufacturers and companies selling the old and new "discoveries." As Dr. Faucher remarked, there is still more known of calf hair and skin than of human hair and skin. And why not? Judging from the allocation of the FDA budget, cosmetics had to make do with $2,470,000, while animal drugs and feeds got $21,789,000.

At a 1982 panel discussion of the New York Society of Security Analysts, Gillette was praised for "risking" $20 million to launch an apricot hull facial scrub. At the same time, "The Rose Sheet" quoted an analyst as saying, "We need to see a fragrance company that is willing to risk $10 or $20 million on a fragrance launch, the way Gillette risked $20 million . . ."

When Dr. Veronica Conley wrote in the American Medical Association's magazine, *Today's Health*, "No other part of the body is so mistreated as the skin," she added, "Physicians echo this statement over and over again as they see patients whose original simple skin condition has been seriously aggravated by self-medication." At the time, she was referring to over-the-counter products for acne and blemishes. Dr. Conley's statement also holds true for some consumers who leap from new "discovery" to a newer and newest "discovery."

In addition to an increasing incidence of dermatitis, more and more dermatologists are seeing acne and blemishes in adults well past adolescence. Many of the skin problems are being traced to cosmetic products.

The FDA has long lists of injury reports from consumers who claim their skins have been adversely affected by various creams and lotions. Among the products accused are some of the most prestigious and well-known names in the cosmetic industry. Price seems to be no criterion. Nor do the "hypoallergenic" labels escape. A review of the yearly lists of complaints indicates a greater number of products of above-average prices, "treatment" products, and a liberal smattering of "hypoallergenics."

The lists also show an increasing number of complaints claiming injuries from various "facial scrubs" or skin-shedding preparations. These have come in the wake of recent heavy promotions of "facial scrubs," which were supposed to scrub away "old and dead skin cells" and reveal "young, new cells," or to "exfoliate," a word embraced by cosmetic copywriters and which, outside the scientific community, more commonly meant "to strip away leaves or bark" rather than to shed skin. In the face of consumer complaints, nature has proved to be a better judge of skin shedding. Evidently, there is a time for snakes and a time for other species.

A few years ago, "peel-off" masks and "masques" were big news, supposedly able to peel off those pesky dead cells and prompt "cell renewal" or get you down to your "new" skin. The FDA still get complaints of injuries from some of these that persist on the market. Another promotion now suggests that you pack imported mud all over your body to rejuvenate yourself at glamorously unmuddy prices.

As the cosmetic companies create new products to get new money to again create "new" products with new prices, the pitch is hauntingly familiar. Meanwhile, no ad or commercial has yet to inform would be cell-shedders that this extraordinary organ we call skin is quite capable of shedding its surplus cells and replacing them with new cells without artificial help. In fact, dermatologists advise washing with mild soap and water followed by a Turkish-toweling as the best way to get rid of any clinging surplus skin cells. A sturdy washcloth also does a creditable job. Conversely, creams and lotions that are not regularly washed off—at least with water—tend to inhibit the normal discarding of surface cells.

According to Dr. Howard T. Behrman, director of dermatological research at New York Medical College, "The younger the woman, the more soap and less cream she should use—the older the woman, the less soap and more cream." Having worked on beauteous luminaries such as Marlene Dietrich, Dr. Behrman's axiom holds true for any gender at any age.

The persistent use of "nourishing" in promoting all types of cosmetics is apparently now tolerated by both the FDA and the FTC who once found the word reason enough to ban an ad or cosmetic from the market.

No matter what is absorbed through the pores, the skin cannot be fed or nourished from the outside in. The skin, like every other part of the body, receives its nourishment from the bloodstream. What you eat and drink for the rest of you is what your skin gets.

Moisturization is another misrepresented and abused banner that is flown from every product from prunes to lipstick. Moisturization in cosmetics began with a professor from Harvard a number of years ago. Dr. Irvin H. Blank of Harvard's Department of Dermatology and its Dermatological Research

Laboratories found that, instead of the skin drawing moisture from the air, as was previously thought in the popular use of glycerin in creams and lotions, a barrier between the skin and the air could keep the skin's own moisture from escaping and thereby keep the skin moist. A barrier could be any occlusive substance such as petroleum jelly, an inexpensive cream or lotion . . . or even an oil from the kitchen.

The professor's theory revolutionized the cosmetic industry—not so much in the products it sold, but in the way it sold those products. Dr. Blank's simple explanation provided the cosmetic industry with the "moisturizer" money umbrella, although products from the beginning of time had been doing the same thing.

When "precious" oils were in vogue a number of years ago, a very expensive "skin nourishing moisturizer" boasted that it contained seven "precious" oils. I asked Dr. Behrman what difference having seven oils instead of one in a cosmetic would make. His reply was: "An oil is an oil. Whether you have one or seven, the effect is the same."

Apart from what you put on your face and body, the best and most effective moisturizer is the water and liquids you put into your body. A dehydrated body is most likely to result in a dehydrated skin. Another help is smoothing a lotion or cream over your body and face while your skin is still wet after washing.

Cosmetic wizardry has yet to produce a cream *at any price* that will do as much as proper attention to good health and cleanliness. A balanced diet, enough exercise, sufficient liquids, avoiding excess sunbathing, and plenty of sleep and relaxation benefit the skin infinitely more than a collection of jars and bottles with designer labels. Beyond that, simple, inexpensive caring and grooming is usually all the normal skin requires.

Despite the extravagant claims calculated to tempt more dollars for psychologically priced potions, no cream has yet been able to stop the clock of aging. If these cosmetic marvels are really effective, why are so many of the personalities who face the motion-picture and television cameras getting so many face lifts?

QUESTIONS AND ANSWERS

I keep being told that mineral oil is not good for the skin—that it robs the skin of vitamins. Is there any truth to this?

I, too, have heard these charges often enough to ask John Wenninger, deputy director of FDA's Division of Cosmetics Technology, about them.

Mr. Wenninger's answer: "We've had several questions from consumers on mineral oil. The questions were phrased in such a way that the consumers wanted to know 'What is harmful about mineral oil in cosmetics?' So we went around and checked.

"There's *no* information that mineral oil in topically applied products is harmful in any respect whatsoever. We asked in one of the letters to consumers, 'What is the *basis* for suspecting that it is?'

"There's nothing in the literature. We talked to the dermatologists and others. *There's nothing in the literature.* And it's absolutely incomprehensible that mineral oil on the skin would extract vitamins. Vitamins are in the bloodstream. Also, topically applied vitamins—there's no evidence that they nourish the body either. *That's a lot of myth and hype.*"

I might point out that the universally used "baby oil" is no more than mineral oil with fragrance—an ingredient with unlisted components that preferably could be left out.

I'm seventeen and have dark, oily skin that still breaks out now and then.

Although you may think your skin is troublesome while you're young, you'll find that your skin will age much less than other skins when you get older. The oil will keep your skin moist and the dark color means that you have more melanin, which is a protective pigment in your skin that will protect it from the harmful rays of the sun that can cause the skin to wrinkle.

In the meantime, wash your face frequently with mild soap and water; stay away from creams or oil-based cosmetics. Check the ingredients. There are water-based foundations if you feel you need to use one. However, most skins such as yours look great without masking them with a foundation. Concentrate on your eyes and mouth and use a powdered blusher if you like.

For your breakouts, try to find a medicated cover that agrees with your skin and doesn't cause other problems. If you still have excess oil, blot it off between washings with a tissue and go over your face with a piece of cotton dipped in witch hazel or a mild astringent, which basically is alcohol with water and fragrance.

At the end of the summer, I tried to get rid of a faded tan and first tried a product that looks like a scouring pad and found it irritated my skin. Then I tried another commercial product that was supposed to remove dead cells. I found it also irritated my skin. Is there something I could use that won't irritate?

There is no guarantee that anything will positively not irritate. Sometimes even water can irritate. It depends on how much you've injured your skin. If your skin is intact, and you want to try a light sloughing, some dermatologists suggest that you wash your face and then go over it with a little plain table salt. Then rinse, and use a simple hand and body lotion on your face to soothe it.

Otherwise, you can use a foundation to even out your tan until your skin is back to its normal color.

I was sold a $15 cream that made my face break out instead of making it moist as I was promised it would. I told the salesgirl about it and she said I could use up the cream on my elbows. I hate to use a $15 cream just for my elbows. What do you think?

I think the sales clerk should have offered you another product or refunded your money. Also, you could have brought your complaint to the manager. If you had not been satisfied at that level, you could have written to the cosmetic company.

No company wants to be responsible for its product harming a consumer; and no consumer should have to pay $15 for a product he or she cannot use.

As a cosmetic merchandiser in one of the country's leading department stores once told me, "A person will return a seventy-nine-cent grocery item to a supermarket with a complaint; why not a cosmetic that may represent a larger investment?"

‾ 18 ‾
Eyes

People will always seek to dramatize and enhance
the most vital of the languages we speak—that of
the eyes.
—Evan Marshall,
Author of *Eye Language*

Eyes—nature's marvel—have caused poets to swoon and lyricists to rhapsodize. Fragile and vulnerable, eyes also have caused most concern in the cosmetic industry. History has not been kind to either the victims or the industry.

Little is known of the injuries that went unreported in the early days of mass-produced cosmetics such as they were. In the 1930s, it was the Lash-Lure blinding of a socialite that prompted the addition of "Cosmetics" to the existing Food and Drug Law.

In 1933, the young socialite was preparing for a formal dinner that was to honor her for her service to the community. During her appointment at the local beauty shop, the hairdresser suggested that she have her eyelashes darkened with Lash Lure, which was being advertised as "The NEW and IMPROVED Eye Brow and Eye Lash Dye."

The woman had to rush to keep another appointment with a photographer; but after the picture-taking, she returned to the shop and had her eyelashes darkened. The before-and-after sketches in the Lash Lure ad were of a model who resembled the attractive brunette; and the appealing "after" sketch, captioned "Radiates Personality," showed the model's lashes dark and thick.

On her way home, the young socialite's eyes began to smart. Within two hours, it became difficult for her to see, but she put in a brief appearance as guest of honor at the dinner. That night, excruciating pain kept her from sleeping. When a doctor examined her in the morning, a swelling rash had appeared on her face and forehead; and her eyes, swollen shut, were being eaten away as though by acid.

Brought to the hospital, she was treated for symptoms as they appeared, but there was no known neutralizing antidote for the synthetic aniline, or coal-tar, dye contained in Lash Lure. A nurse's terse professional notes recorded the woman's agony as Lash Lure's dye destroyed her eyeballs.

A month later, the socialite, blinded and disfigured, sat for another photograph in her own tragic before-and-after Lash Lure sequence. Her "after" photograph bore no resemblance to Lash Lure's advertised promise.

The blinding occurred on May 17, 1933, and Lash Lure no longer is on the market. But the young woman's lifelong tragedy was only indirectly responsible for Lash Lure's removal from the market *five years after her blinding*. Although the *Journal of the American Medical Association* reported multiple injuries caused by Lash Lure in addition to those sustained by the socialite, the eyelash dye continued to be advertised and sold throughout most of the country.

Newspapers, benefiting from Lash Lure's advertising, neglected to inform their readers of the consequences suffered by some of Lash Lure's users. Almost a year after the blinding, the dye claimed another victim. A beautician began to darken the brows and lashes of her fifty-two-year-old mother with Lash Lure, but the reaction was so instantaneous and severe that the daughter didn't get beyond "beautifying" one eye. After eight days of violent illness, her mother died.

Since then, there have been eye injuries from insufficiently tested dandruff shampoos, contaminated mascara, a permanent-wave neutralizer, and eyeliners containing coal-tar dye forbidden for use around the eyes since the 1938 passage of the Food, Drug, and Cosmetic Act. In addition, there are continuous reports of allergic reactions to eye shadows, including those promoted as being hypo-allergenic.

In November 1981, a surprising number of beauty salons were promoting eyelash dyeing, when a New York City doctor suspected that the dye being used might have coal-tar dye similar to the dye that had blinded the socialite in 1933. He sent a sample of the dye to the New York district of the FDA, where an analysis confirmed the doctor's suspicion.

The dye was Dr. Olbrich's Combinal Dye for Eyebrows/Eyelashes, imported from W. Pauli, a company in Vienna, Austria, and distributed by Dynex International, Ltd. of New York City. Intended primarily for professional use, the dye apparently lacked ingredient listing, prompting the analysis.

At the request of the New York City district of the FDA, New York state authorities embargoed the 3,057 quarter-ounce tubes of Dr. Olbrich's eyebrow and eyelash dye in the Dynex warehouse. The 3,057 tubes were enough to dye 100,000 pairs of eyelashes.

About the same time the New York doctor was having his suspected sample analyzed, the Los Angeles district of the FDA received a complaint from a woman in Fremont, California, who claimed to have suffered erosion of her left cornea after a beautician had applied the dye to her lashes. Fortunately, she escaped permanent vision loss.

On April 9, 1982, five months after the reports, FDA in Washington decided to alert the public through a press release. FDA warned that Dr. Olbrich's Combinal dyes for eyelashes and eyebrows were nationally distributed in black, brown, gray, and blue shades, and that they contained coal-tar ingredients that might cause permanent injury to the eyes, including blindness.

The agency also cautioned the beauty salons and their customers not to use the products, and issued an import alert to prevent the further importation of the dyes. According to the FDA, Dynex was recalling its products from its customers.

On November 8, 1982, a year after the New York and California reports, FDA issued a revised Import Alert. Dr. Olbrich was not alone. Other eyelash dyes found to contain the forbidden coal tar were: all shades of Andora, manufactured by Andora-Cosmetic, Vienna, Austria; Refecto Cil in graphite, black, brown, blue, and gray, manufactured by Gschwenter-Haar Kosmetic Products, also of Vienna; Henna Gora in black, brown, and blue-black, manufactured by Else Sperlich Chem. Kosm. Fabrick, Berlin, East Germany; Permalash in black and brown, distributed by Faces Enterprises, Ltd., Baltimore, Maryland, and manufactured by Zena Cosmetic Co., London, England; and Continental Eyelash and Eyebrow Dye in black and brown, imported and distributed by Lon's Cosmetics, Brooklyn, New York.

Three of the six brands became the subject of an FDA recall in 1982. The agency's field compliance branches were told to alert the local postal inspectors and U.S. customs agents to the possible entry of the six dyes, to collect samples for analysis, and to hold the shipments in their custody pending examination "due to the severe health hazard of this product."

Unfortunately, all this was after many more than Dr. Olbrich's 100,000 applications to possible victims were discovered to be scattered throughout the country.

Since few consumers will see the Import Alert, and recalls seldom are complete, stragglers may persist in the market for years with unaware beauticians offering to dye client's eyelashes to do away with the "bother of putting on mascara every day." In the interest of safety, the FDA explanation of the dangerous coal-tar dyes bears repeating.

> The products are believed to be widely distributed in the United States, although they probably are not sold for direct use by consumers, but rather sold to and used in beauty salons. Before use, the products are mixed with hydrogen peroxide and applied by a beautician to the eyelashes with a cotton swab. The primary distributors in the U.S. are likely to be firms that supply goods to beauty salons; however, it may also be shipped directly to beauty salons by the manufacturer.

Consumers who buy from stores that specialize in products for professional use and beauty salons should be especially careful in their buying, since cosmetics intended for professional use are not required to list ingredients and usually do not have adequate directions for use, if they have any at all.

Eye makeup has become almost mandatory in recent years. Revlon boasts it has more than 150 shades of eye shadow. Practically every Sunday newspaper is splashed with ads heralding another clutch of mascaras, eyeliners, eyebrow pencils, and eye shadows. Fashion magazines devote pages to "the new eyes" and more pages telling readers how to achieve them with half a dozen prerequisites. And although the most famous of the makeup artists, including Pablo Manzoni who for many years was known as Pablo of Elizabeth Arden, suggest neutral shadows for eyelids, every street still yields a parade of surrealistic bright blue or green eyelids seemingly floating disembodied from reticent faces.

Amidst all this have come questions with few answers and demands without solutions. Notoriety has come to the Draize Eye Test, accompanied with misunderstanding and calculated misdirection.

The Draize Eye Test is named after Dr. John Draize, an FDA pharmacologist and the principle author of a 1944 paper that provided a numerical scale in determining the degree of irritancy of a tested substance. Rarely mentioned is another Draize Test—the Draize 24-hour Patch Test, which tests substances for skin adverse reactions. Both tests use rabbits.

When I met Dr. Draize a number of years ago, I found him to be much like a kindly family doctor, unassuming and sincere in his efforts to protect consumers from untested products whose potential for harm was unknown.

When the Draize Eye Test was introduced in 1944, cosmetics not only required no testing but did not have to disclose ingredients. And with the country enmeshed in World War II, cosmetics could not have been of great, if any, concern to Dr. Draize or the FDA. According to reports, Dr. Draize evolved the test as part of the war effort to protect our soldiers.

Yet, in 1980, when the Draize Eye Test was selected for public focus, the cosmetic industry became the target of demonstrations and Revlon was selected for picketing. The Draize Eye Test became the Draize Rabbit Blinding Test. Circulars were distributed with photographs of grotesquely injured rabbit eyes. The printed sheet, however, was headed "Federal Hazardous Substances Act Regulations," from which cosmetics are exempt, and was from the U.S. Consumer Product Safety Commission, from which cosmetics also escaped. The unidentified photographs, therefore, were unlikely those of cosmetic tests.

During a telephone interview before the beginning of the demonstrations and advertising, I asked for documentation of the charge that those in the cosmetic industry were blinding rabbits. There was none.

Since I've been monitoring the industry and examining its shortcomings for twenty-five years, I explained that any cosmetic that would be caustic enough to blind a rabbit should not even be considered to the point of being tested. If there were such cosmetics, I wanted to know about them. None were produced.

I then spent a number of hours giving a minicourse in cosmetics, which apparently fell on deadened ears. When I asked why the attacks weren't directed against the household cleaning products that were more apt to be caustic and cause damage to rabbit eyes during testing, I received no reply.

Later it was admitted that focusing on cosmetics and claiming they were blinding rabbits had been deliberate, the facts bent to evoke a stronger public reaction.

Representatives of various groups appeared on radio and television to repeat misinformation. When a visiting head of a national organization again told radio listeners that the government required cosmetic companies to test their products and to do dire things to rabbit eyes before marketing cosmetics, I called the local chapter to arrange an interview. I told a local representative that I was sympathetic to the cause of diminishing the use of animals used in testing and seeking alternate tests, but that I also thought it would be helpful if the information being given was factual.

Since there was to be an organized march on Washington, I offered to go along to interview the principals and to report on their activities. I was told I would be called by another member to make arrangements. When I did not receive a call and the departure was imminent, I called, only to encounter shouting hostility and a receiver banged in my ear.

What is the Draize Eye Test? Briefly quoting from the procedure:

> The animal is held firmly but gently until quiet. The test material is placed in one eye of each animal by gently pulling the lower lid away from the eyeball to form a cup into which the test substance is dropped. The lids are then gently held together for one second and the animal is released. The other eye remaining untreated, serves as a control. For testing liquids .01 milliliter is used.

Stories of animals being tortured to produce another shampoo swept the land. Pickets marched protesting the blindings of rabbits on the steps of the wrong industry. Boycotts were begun. And Revlon struck a bargain.

In December 1980, Revlon announced that it was establishing a research program at Rockefeller University to find alternatives to the Draize Eye Test. Revlon provided $750,000 for a three-year program under the guidance of Dr. Dennis M. Stark, director of the Laboratory Animal Research and associate professor. It was an easier route than charging slander and attracting even more attention. It dissolved the picket lines, broke the boycott, and garnered more than its weight in healing publicity.

The CTFA and its member companies followed Revlon's example, in September 1981, with a $1 million grant to establish The Johns Hopkins Center for Alternatives to Animal Testing, at the Johns Hopkins University School of Hygiene and Public Health in Baltimore, Maryland. The program, headed by Dr. Alan M. Goldberg, has since received additional funding from Bristol-Myers and the Geraldine R. Dodge Foundation.

Both programs have made promising starts, but at the end of 1983, the Draize Eye Test remains the only test for eye irritancy, although some companies have made refinements in the technique. At the end of 1983, one promising refinement from the research program at Rockefeller University is ready for outside testing.

The "blind bunny" ads that appeared in *The New York Times* did prompt a new awareness that too many animals were being needlessly sacrificed in testing laboratories. It had been an awareness, not only of the general public and the animal protectionists, but of those doing the testing, that had been growing for a number of years, if not decades.

As Dr. Grover V. Foster, Jr., chairman of the CTFA Test Systems Review Task Force, explained, "Internationally, the concern for animal rights was spearheaded by antivivisectionists in the United Kingdom ... which had as its objective the development of humane research techniques."

The movement, begun in 1969, evolved into the generally accepted rule known as the "three Rs"—*Replacement, Reduction, and Refinement of Experiments on Live Animals.*

Although there have been some replacements—most notably, the test for pregnancy, which no longer uses rabbits; and the Ames test for mutagenicity—there has been greater progress in refinement of tests and reduction of the animals used. For instance, a 1978 National Institutes of Health survey of laboratory animals in the United States showed that, from 1968 through 1978, there had been a 40-percent reduction in the number of laboratory animals acquired.

Although the "blinded rabbit" campaign used questionable means to attract attention, it did spur the cosmetic industry into defending itself by funding additional and accelerated efforts to find alternatives to undesirable as well as time- and cost-consuming testing methods. *The New York Times* ad with the reportedly staged "blinded bunny" photograph also attracted the attention of Dr. Dennis Stark.

Dr. Stark, a veterinarian with a Ph.D. in immunochemistry, virology, and biochemistry, and intensely dedicated to research, was intrigued by the challenge of finding an alternative to the objective and subjective Draize Test.

The plan for a research program devoted to finding alternatives for the Draize was formulated over dinner with a fellow veterinarian during the pillorying of Revlon. With his background and knowledge of animals, Dr. Stark was uniquely qualified to head the program.

"So we wrote Revlon," Dr. Stark said, "and indicated that if they had any interest, we would be willing to do some studies for them."

After discussions, Revlon agreed to fund the program at Rockefeller University with the $750,000. When I commented that he had, therefore, been instrumental in thinking of the plan, Dr. Stark admitted with a chuckle, "Yes, I will state that categorically. But then, again, we'd said, 'Here's the potential.'"

Then, retreating into modesty, Dr. Stark added, "Well, I had the idea. Whether or not I transmitted that idea and it passed up to the powers that be there, I don't know."

However it happened, it was a brilliant public relations coup that promises to bear future fruit, although Dr. Stark believes that it will take a number of procedures rather than merely one alternative test to take the place of the Draize Eye Test.

Meanwhile, fringe cosmetic companies are profiting from the public perception that the larger companies are blinding rabbits to test cosmetics. *They*, they tell would-be consumers, *do not blind rabbits by using the Draize Test.* What they're not saying is that many of them are not doing *any* testing.

Also, what is not realized is that the eye irritation test is a small part of cosmetic safety testing . . . and eyes can be dam-

EYES **199**

aged by more than irritation. Most routine testing requires no animals—tests, for instance, for purity, alkalinity, contamination, inflammability, combustibility, microbial content, and mutagenicity.

Eye makeup, such as Lash Makeup in black and brown by Rorer, Intl. Cosmetics Ltd., was recalled because of bacterial contamination. Studio Girl Black Brush-on Mascara by Studio Girl Cosmetics., Inc. was found to be contaminated with *pseudomonas aeruginosa,* a pathogenic bacteria that can blind.

Also found to be contaminated with *pseudomonas aeruginosa* were: Avon Skinplicity Moisturizer AM/PM; Eucerin Moisture Formula by Beiersdorf Inc.; Medissage II Lotion; Hospital Care Lotion and Hospital Skin Lotion by A. R. Williams & Co. Inc. and repacked by S/P Industries; Revlon Milk Plus 6 24-Hour Face Moisturizer; Ultra Feminine Cream by Helena Rubinstein, Inc.; Cattier Mineral Shampoo Moussargile for Oily Hair and Cattier Mineral Shampoo Moussargile for Dry Hair by Pierre Cattier Ltd., New York, N.Y. Clarity Super Cleaner by General Chemical and Cosmetics, a subsidiary of Germaine Monteil, New York, N.Y., was contaminated with *pseudomonas putida,* a less virulent bacteria.

Many more cosmetics were found to be bacterially contaminated. Others contained nonpermitted color additives. None of these would have done eyes any good if they had found their way there. All could be tested for bacteria and nonpermitted color additives without using a single animal.

Do cosmetics need to be tested? You bet they do. Do they have to be? Not at all. Are they? Don't bet on it. Are we ready to turn our backs on the use of animals in research and testing? And can we disregard animal testing as a gauge for human beings? One scientist reminded us that *man is an animal.*

Also, it may come as a shock to know, as Dr. Stark pointed out, that in 1981, human beings were a not-too-distant second to rats as the most frequently used "research animals" in experimental medicine. Mice were a close third; dogs were well down the list; then came the rabbit at about 5 percent; a couple of other species were, along with the cat, about 2 percent; and lastly, the pig, at about 1 percent. The human beings involved in basic research are in addition to countless numbers who become the "research animals'" in final resolutions of drugs and other products and the innumerable consumer panels throughout the world.

Don Davis, *Drug & Cosmetic Industry* editor, critical of the tactics used by the animal protectionists, suggested that the pathetic photographs of the rabbits "obviously were designed to generate the same sort of propaganda appeal those 1914 posters of Belgian babies impaled on German bayonets had for the noncommitted nations." Conceding the points won by the animal protection lobby, he warned that "the search for an Ames-type test for assaying the irritation potential of a cosmetic chemical still looks no closer than three years away."

According to the trade magazine editor, since finding animal models that accurately duplicate human skin was difficult, the overwhelming problem of finding a nonanimal model of the eye needed "a quantum step . . . before we can talk realistically about using a nonhuman, nonanimal model to predict eye irritation, skin penetration, or metabolic effects on animal or human host."

As for achieving complete elimination of the animal population in cosmetic (or drug) laboratories, Mr. Davis quoted Dr. A. Clifford Barger of the Harvard University Medical School. Dr. Barger told the school's medical forum: "Ultimately, you can't prevent blindness in bacteria, which don't have eyes. You can't treat blood pressure in tissue cultures, which don't have heart or blood vessels. You can't relieve arthritis in protozoa, which don't have bones or joints. To study such common and often devastating disorders, researchers have no choice but to work at least some of the time with animals that have relevant organs. Nor can surgery such as organ transplants or reattachment of severed limbs be perfected without animal trials."

QUESTIONS AND ANSWERS

How can I learn more about animal testing in relation to cosmetics?

CTFA has printed a brochure on "Animal Testing and Human Safety" and has agreed to make it available to the public on request. For a copy, write to The Cosmetic, Toiletry and Fragrance Association, Inc., 1110 Vermont Avenue, N.W., Suite 800, Washington, D.C. 20005.

For all the other questions I've received on cosmetics and animal testing, I defer to Ann Landers and repeat an answer she gave to one of her readers:

A great deal of propaganda, accompanied by heartbreaking photographs, has ignited a campaign to halt the alleged cruelty to animals in research laboratories. But before you get out your crying towels (and checkbooks), folks, here are some facts:

Some animal lovers have gone so far as to suggest that prisoners and elderly patients be used instead of animals. Add to that bizarre notion the fact that 13 million dogs and cats were destroyed in shelters last year because no one wanted them. Yet thousands of well-heeled organizations are trying to stop the use of animals in medical research laboratories. I ask you, does this make sense?

Animals housed in universities, medical schools, hospitals and research centers are monitored by the U.S. Department of Agriculture. Periodic surprise inspection visits are conducted under the Animal Welfare Act. The National Institutes of Health have standards governing such experimentation for all scientists who receive NIH funds. Animals' quarters must meet space specifications, be air-conditoned and kept clean. Potentially painful experiments must be done under anesthesia.

Animal experimentation made it possible to immunize millions of children, all over the world, against polio, diphtheria, mumps, measles, hepatitis, etc. Add to that list every person who receives an antibiotic to fight infection, insulin for diabetes, anti-inflammatory agents for arthritis, chemotherapy for cancer, medication to control hypertension and drugs for the treatment of mental illness. Every person who has undergone the replacement of a joint, or the reattachment of a severed finger or limb, kidney dialysis, heart surgery or organ transplantation owes a debt to animal experimentation. Pet lovers should be aware that the progress made in veterinary medicine is due largely to experiments on animals.

There has been a decline of approximately 50% in the use of animals for laboratory testing since 1968 due to the development of highly sophisticated test-tube techniques, but experiments involving the heart and the brain cannot be performed in test tubes. They must be conducted with live tissue.

No person in his right mind wants to see an animal suffer, but until the day comes when all medical problems are solved we must experiment with animals. So let's hear it for the dogs that went to Harvard. They may well have made a more meaningful contribution to humanity than some people we know."

Don Davis, editor of *Drug & Cosmetic Industry,* ended an editorial with: "Each of us is a consumer concerned about obtaining the ultimate assurance of safety in those products we purchase and use. With present-day technology, if the cost of achieving such assurance mandates the sacrifice of an occasional hairless mouse or rabbit or laboratory rat, then it is a price that we are prepared to pay. It is a delusion and a sham at this point to say we can achieve one without the other."

— 19 —
Keeping Clean and Smelling Good

The average American places 10 to 40 pounds of
soaps, toiletries and cosmetics on his or her skin
annually.
—**Dr. Robert J. Scheuplein,**
Food and Drug Administration

The American proclivity for brushing after meals,
daily bathing, showering, shaving, deodorizing, and routinely
shampooing, manicuring, and sunbathing fills our homes with
cosmetic staples. As products constantly used in and on our
bodies, these staples should meet government standards, safeguards, and checks similar to those applicable to food and
drugs. Since they are not required to, they don't.

However, since we've become too accustomed to dry
armpits and talcumed babies to do without cosmetic staples,
and neither Congress nor the FDA seems willing to rock the
status quo, our only recourse is to attempt to choose and use
these staples judiciously and defensively.

Take dry armpits, for instance. The stores shelve a bewildering array of deodorants and antiperspirants in an even

more bewildering number of forms and packages. The aerosol spray is the least economical and the most questionable, leaving one to wonder why the industry still produces them. Of all the forms—solid, roll-on, liquid, cream, and saturated pads— the aerosol delivers the least product at the greatest cost.

Apart from the reports, in 1974, of aerosols damaging the atmosphere, consumer groups informed an FDA panel of experts that the zirconium being used in antiperspirant aerosols could be causing malignant tumors. The panel then voted to recommend that those aerosols be removed from the market.

Action was stayed when Procter & Gamble, producers of Super Dry Sure and Dry Formula Secret, both zirconium-containing aerosols, asked to meet with the panel and present its case for continuing the aerosols. The FDA then found itself in the middle of not only consumer-group pressure supported by its own expert panel to take the aerosols off the market, but an intra-industry fight as well.

More than a year before the panel's recommendation, Gillette had voluntarily recalled its newly marketed Extra Strength Right Guard and Soft & Dri when tests on monkeys showed mild lung inflammation that implicated zirconyl salts used in Gillette's aerosols.

Gillette's action prompted its competitor, Procter & Gamble—with a major investment in its Super Dry Sure and Dry Formula Secret zirconyl-containing aerosols—to rush to reassure FDA and others who might be considering putting its products into the endangered category. By so doing, it gained a stay of *years* while Washington pondered and examined P&G's justification. In the meantime, P&G and others, including Carter, producer of Arrid XXX, continued to produce and market the suspected zirconium aerosols.

On June 5, 1975, almost two years after Gillette had voluntarily recalled its products and seven months after the panel recommendation, the FDA announced that, lacking proof of absolute safety, it would consider zirconium-containing antiperspirant aerosols to be unapproved new drugs and, therefore, not marketable.

It took another two years before FDA finally ruled zirconium to be a "deleterious substance that may render a cosmetic aerosol product that contains it injurious to users." As for the consumers—unless they had access to the trade press and the *Federal Register*—how could they know that "When used in aerosol form, some zirconium will reach the deep portions of the lungs of users"? Or that "Evidence indicates that certain zirconium compounds have caused human skin granulomas [inflammatory tumors or growths] and toxic effects in the lung and other organs of experimental animals." Or that "Unlike the skin, the lung will not reveal the presence of granulomatous changes until they have become advanced and, in some cases, permanent." Or note the consistency with which the delayed FDA actions, if they came, were arthritic *reactions* to outside sources and forces.

One of the most incriminating reports of aerosol deodorant sprays causing lung damage was that from a Denver hospital that found both a physical therapist and her roommate to be suffering from fibrous lesions in their lungs that were diagnosed as sarcoidosis. The cause of the lesions puzzled the examining doctors until they learned that the two young women had used the same brand of deodorant spray.

Later, ten otherwise healthy men developed similar symptoms after using two brands of deodorant spray, one of which was the same as that used by the women. The deodorant sprays were then sprayed at guinea pigs. All the animals developed lung lesions.

The trend in marketing and consumer buying has been steadily away from deodorant and antiperspirant aerosols in the United States, while Europe still clings more tenaciously to the aerosols. Considering that it is the easily reachable armpits that are to be kept dry or odor free, even from the standpoint of economy it seems wasteful, if not risky, to spray the air around the armpits rather than using something directly in them. Currently, the best bet seems to be the solid stick. It's nonmessy, easily controlled, travels well, and, comparatively, is the best ounce-for-ounce value.

At the turn of the seventh decade of the twentieth century, the cosmetic industry discovered another part of the human body to deodorize with aerosol sprays. The land was visited by crotch sprays.

Most publicized and advertised were the "feminine hygiene" sprays, although gynecologists and others advised that soap and water were much better "feminine hygiene." Less publicized were the "masculine hygiene" sprays, which were labeled "a refreshing deodorizing spray for very personal parts" and available in a choice of berry, lime, lemon, and natural. Then, of course, there was Charles Revson's Pub "Below the Belt Deodorant Spray ... a deodorizing men's powder spray for the groin area."

As the reports of injuries from the sprays accumulated, Dr. Francis N. Marzulli, FDA's chief of dermatoxicology, said, "I certainly would like a plug for people using soap and water instead of using all this. If you take a bath, you'll have more cleanliness than you do by putting a bunch of chemicals on the various and sundry parts."

After reading in gynecology journals that 40 to 60 percent of women using the crotch spray reported discomfort and itching, one woman wrote to the editor of *Advertising Age* suggesting another use for the sprays. "Aim for the cockroaches," she wrote; "it *works*."

The piecemeal approach brings to mind a show-stopping poster at a cosmetic trade exhibition. It showed a misty photograph of a nude female figure, her arms at her sides, standing straight and looking as though she were facing a firing squad. Reminiscent of the familiar butcher-shop illustrations identifying the various cuts of beef on an animal, the various parts of the woman's body were labeled: "Her Hair," "Her Face," "Her Body," "Her Legs," "Her Arms," "Her Feet." The poster was captioned: *"What we won't think of next is what someone else thought of last week."*

Although her crotch was clearly visible, it was unlabeled. Apparently someone else had thought of crotch sprays, and their producers had collected almost $60 million from susceptible women in the previous year. Instead of getting the fulfillment of Madison Avenue's leering promises for their money and trouble, thousands of women got painful, lacerated, and irritated crotches.

I asked Dr. Marzulli if he'd had any reports from those using the male sprays, but none had reached him at the time. However, graphic examples of photosensitization from perfumes exposed to sunlight and the resultant long-term skin discolorations shown at an American Medical Association conference, may have been clues to the evolution of crotch sprays.

According to Dr. Adolph Rostenberg, Jr., one young woman dabbed perfume around her ears and on her cheek, went out into the sun, and developed a partially brown ear and a large brown patch on her cheek. Another woman had a brown neck and a mottled chest with brown rivulets between her breasts, which Dr. Rostenberg explained had come from being "a bit more greedy about splashing on her perfume."

Another woman "must have dumped herself right in the bottle, and there was very extensive involvement."

The last slide showed a man with a browned, swollen, and very irritated penis. "He apparently wanted to perfume himself all over."

The current cost of designer-name perfumes being introduced at a revolving-door rate may be curtailing the generous use of the past. Not too long ago, thirty-five dollars an ounce for big-name perfumes was considered to be costly. Now every week sees a multimillion-dollar hullabaloo about a "new perfume" from famous or semiobscure designers, movie stars, and sundry personalities, at $130 and $140 an ounce. For a wink of an eye, there was even a line of fragrances named for an author who had become famous for turning out hundreds of candy-box romantic novels.

The trade press clucks its tongue at the madness and points to losses as it monitors line after line being sold and bought or swallowed or forgotten. The "noses" in the big fragrance houses that supply the perfumes to which designer names are attached are delighted to work overtime. Less well-known companies begin lines of copies, facsimile, or "like" perfumes that mimic the famous names at fractional prices, and are battled as invaders by the producers for the snob set.

The favorable exchange of the dollar overseas has nurtured a new industry that's busily diverting shipments of big-name perfumes, intended for parts other than the United States. The perfumes are then sold here at substantial discounts. This has disturbed the big-namers, intent on preserving the mystique of psychological pricing, into pressuring law-enforcing authorities and any other authorities into Keystone-Cop chasing after the cheeky culprits.

According to CTFA's Ed Kavanaugh: "We have two problems, mainly in the fragrance area, but also coming into the cosmetic area. One involves counterfeiting which is becoming a very serious problem for this industry. And the other is diversion of products.

"Because of the strong dollar and the weak French franc, that product is being diverted out of France at such a cheap price that . . . even though it's [the U.S. company's] product, they're underselling themselves because we have a black market occurring with those products being diverted out of France."

I wondered if the fragrance companies weren't doing it to themselves with their clockwork introduction of new perfumes at $130 an ounce. Maybe outsiders were catching on to psychological pricing and finding that consumers were as responsive, if not more responsive, to psychological *downward* pricing. Even in these days of inflated prices, $130 still buys a lot of hamburger.

But hold on—yet another new perfume has joined the horde. The October 1983 issue of the trade magazine *Soap/Cosmetics/Chemical Specialities* announced: "Balenciaga's new 'Prelude,' launched in France last year . . . is priced at $100 for 1/2 ounce."

Since the late, great designer most likely had nothing to do with creating "Prelude," one wonders if he would have been shocked or delighted to know that a perfume was tagged at $200 an ounce on the strength of his name.

Two hundred dollars for an ounce of perfume? *That's a lot of psychology in a very small bottle.*

QUESTIONS AND ANSWERS

What is the difference between a deodorant and an antiperspirant?

The words tell the meaning. A deodorant *deodorizes* without promising to stop perspiration or to stop "wetness." An antiperspirant promises to stop perspiration or literally is *against perspiration.* Many antiperspirants are labeled as antiperspirant-deodorants, which combines the two meanings, but if there's no perspiration, there's usually no odor.

I would like to use some of the famous but expensive perfumes, but I can't afford the prices. Any suggestions?

If you're lucky enough to come upon samples, grab them. Sometimes there are gifts with purchases. If you can combine your purchase with your own gift-giving or with something you actually need, then you're ahead; but watch out that you're not tempted to overspend just to get the gift.

If all else fails, see if they have a small-size package of bath oil in that fragrance. The bath oil usually costs a good deal less than the perfume, and a drop or two, dabbed where it will not stain clothing, will make you smell of the expensive perfume and will last almost as long. A drop or two smoothed on hair also should do no harm and get the message to the noses around and above you.

If there's no bath oil in the fragrance, try the smallest size of cologne or toilet water. Usually the cologne or toilet water is potent enough to wear and is less likely to evaporate before you use it up.

Whatever you buy, the liquid in a plain bottle will give you more for your money than the sprays that dissipate the fragrance in the air around you. Also look for sales. Often, even the biggest names are on sale for special promotions.

I've seen a number of stores that specialize in perfumes and colognes that are supposed to be copies of the popular high-priced perfumes. Are they worth buying?

If you like the way they smell and the price is low enough to compensate for their not being the real thing, and perhaps being a bit weaker in concentration, I see no reason to pass them up. Wearing a fragrance is not like wearing a piece of apparel on which the designer has managed to put his name or identifying mark and, thereby, seduced the buyer into doing his advertising for him.

I'd rather chance a reasonably priced fragrance that

suits me and doesn't pretend to be other than it is than chance buying a counterfeit famous-name fragrance on a street corner or in a store with a questionable reputation.

Also, if you check the stores, you'll still find some old favorites that are no longer heavily advertised and therefore have managed to keep their prices within reason. There's a big plus in the fact that they've remained in the market over the years while a multitude of newcomers have disappeared almost as quickly as they appeared.

20
Growing
Older

Who well lives, long lives; for this age of ours
Should not be numbered by years, daies, and
hours.
—Guillaume de Salluste,
Seigneur du Bartas

In 1983, the "older woman" was discovered in the never-never land of entertainment. Supplanting the 1960s cry of the young to "never trust anyone over thirty," a mutual admiration society declared it was *chic* to be over forty in the 1980s. It may have been mere coincidence that many of the 1960s young had ripened into fashionable forties by 1983.

Articles appeared throughout the nation extolling the charms of over-forty motion-picture and television stars. Legendary stars, formerly dismissed as being "over the hill" and put out to pasture, were recalled to appear on television. To the apparent amazement of executives in charge, some of whom had not been born when the stars were at their zenith, ratings rose and skyrocketed. Barbara Stanwyck, well past forty, walked off with an Emmy and stole the Emmy show itself.

An assembly line of books by over-forty stars and personalities telling their "secrets" of beauty and exercise were published in a space of months. There were records and tapes and exercise franchises. Soon the beauty, exercise, and "fitness" craze swept in some under-forties, male and female.

Harper's Bazaar devoted its September issue to "OVER-40 & LOVING IT!" The cover featured Elizabeth Taylor, fifty-one, in makeup and a photograph that lost Elizabeth Taylor along the way.

"Over-forty" has become the cliché that's used to describe every older woman. Rarely, if ever, is a man described as being "over-forty." For women it is the unspeakable abyss in editorial and promotional thrusts—even though those perpetuating the cliché may be well over forty.

But yes, Virginia, there *are* women over fifty as well as over forty. There are even women over sixty and seventy and eighty and some over ninety and maybe a few over a hundred—decades over forty, and a goodly number to whom forty was merely mid-life. These have been the truly forgotten women.

According to government surveys, 60 percent of the elderly in the country are women. Of them, 15 million women are over the age of sixty-five, and 3.5 million over eighty.

On October 25, 1983, 400 delegates from various women's and elder women's interest groups met in New York City to discuss their problems in the New York State Conference on Midlife and Older Women.

Judy Klemesrud of *The New York Times* reported New York Representative Geraldine A. Ferraro as saying: "Gray hair and wrinkles give a man authority, dignity, and importance. They give a woman reason to rush out for hair dye and a face lift. As a result, many women deny their age, and by doing so perpetuate the myth that older women have nothing useful to contribute to American life.

"It's high time to lay this little old lady syndrome to rest."

On the other hand, Bernard Meltzer, who has a large following on his call-in radio program broadcast daily from Station WOR in New York, counsels the many women callers threatened with age discrimination and prejudice to shave their ages whenever necessary. In other words, if a woman doesn't look an age as it is perceived to look, why not meet the perception?

If confronted by a birth certificate or the need to prove you've lived beyond the age when you're ready to begin collecting social security, you can always revert to quoting Oscar Wilde. "One should never trust a woman who tells one her real age," he warned. "A woman who would tell one that, would tell one anything."

At the same time the delegates were meeting in New York to adopt a fifty-plank "action agenda" in the hope of affecting legislation in Washington, the CTFA was holding a scientific regulatory conference in Washington and taking note of the need for more work on producing products for the elder set.

To catch up with the graying of America, responsible members of the cosmetic industry must race hard and work even harder to sustain the claims being made for some of their products and to justify the prices being charged.

For a very long time, government regulators and legislators also have ignored the abuses in some of the claims being made for products calculated to tempt dollars from susceptible would-be believers, many of whom are elderly and slim of purse. Newspapers and periodicals—some of them eager for any advertising—carry ads promising youth in a bottle or a jar at $20, $30, and $40 with "testimonials" that tell of use "forever after."

Many of the ads focus on the "60-" or "90-second face

lift" or "how to look 15 years younger." Headlines promise
"face lifts without surgery," or challenge you to prove that the
persons pictured have had face lifts even though, in some
cases, the persons look as old as or older than their ages.
Mailboxes are being stuffed with bulky envelopes of direct mail pieces, replete with "testimonials" from seventy- and
eighty-year-old "satisfied users." Some urge would-be partak-
ers of the fountain of youth to order the "economy" size and
save handling charges. The "economy" size runs to well over
$100.

The "quick face lift" products are a reprise of $25-an-
ounce temporary wrinkle removers of the mid-1960s. Before-
and-after photographs showed a wrinkled face emerging
smooth and clear after the claimed magic of the "wrinkle re-
mover."

At the counters, consumers were at a loss to find a demonstrator vial to try before buying. I found one in Paris and
dabbed a bit of the fluid at the corner of my eyes. Sure enough,
it tightened the skin as egg white would. As it dried, it also
crumbled and flaked like dried egg white. No appreciable
smoothing survived normal skin movement.

The 1960s "wrinkle removers" were based on protein
serum from cattle blood supplied by slaughterhouses. In an
FDA conflict as to whether these should be considered drugs or
cosmetics, various companies dragged the conflict through the
courts for a number of years. Then the FTC was roused to discover that the before-and-after photographs were not as advertised.

For a while there were special sales—and even a package for any males who wanted to try the magic. Packages were
reduced to one-fifth the original price and finally disappeared
from the counters.

In the 1980s, the new crop is pushing collagen, a gelatinous substance found in connective tissue. It's *animal protein,* and where does it come from?

Other youth "miracles" claim they'll give you "serious skin treatment" with not only collagen but placenta extracts and rare herbs. So, back we go to the cattle, this time for the placenta or afterbirth thrown into slop pails after the birth of a calf.

Whatever constituents of value there are in the placentas go to the pharmaceutical manufacturers. The inert residue goes to any cosmetic company that will take it.

Because the placenta or placental extracts used in cosmetics have been found to be inert, the FDA long ago forbade making any claims for placenta on labeling although cosmetic manufacturers may use the ingredient and feature it on the label. Since most claims are made in advertising, which usually sails safely by the FTC, placenta pushers count on the ads propelling the hopeful consumer into buying the product in a store, or more likely, filling out the coupon that usually accompanies the ad, and sending the money through the mail without seeing or reading the label.

As for the unidentified "rare and exotic herbs," one manufacturer told me flatly there were *no* rare ingredients used in cosmetics.

"The things we need," he said, "are in abundant supply or can be reproduced inexpensively. The *freaks* [exotic ingredients] are usually those which have been on the shelf because they have no usefulness."

Not all claims that test credibility are made by obscure or post-office-box companies. Some claims made by some famous-name companies so annoy some famous-name competitors that they have been known to bring their annoyances to regulatory agencies.

In a backlash to deregulation, which was supposed to help the industry, members of the cosmetic community are grumbling about how deregulation and executive orders have dismembered the Federal Trade Commission, which is supposed to listen to complaints about competitor's claims being made in advertising, and crumpled the Food and Drug Administration, which is supposed to listen to complaints of contested claims on labeling.

At one time, companies that felt their competitors were taking unfair advantage by making claims with questionable proof could complain to the agencies nested in Washington and have some assurance that some reprimanding action might be taken. With the Washington referees chilled by the cold wind of executive orders, the complaining competitors have been driven to take their briefs to the Better Business Bureau (BBB) like lowly consumers. Still, since the BBB is funded by business, why not nudge BBB's National Advertising Division (NAD) into taking a look at the offending claims?

As *The Rose Sheet* of F-D-C Reports reported, an unnamed "leading competitor" and a college professor brought one of the most famous names, Estée Lauder, to NAD's attention. A cosmetic watcher would have noted that, in 1982, Estée Lauder was energetically advertising and promoting Swiss Performing Extract at $12.50 for 7/8 of an ounce, promising "Its amazing capabilities can help your skin look better *instantly*." Among other claims, Swiss Performing Extract promised to perform *"24 hours a day."*

By 1983, Swiss Performing ads had given way to Age-Controlling Creme, at $20 for half an ounce, and Night Repair, at $35 for .87 of an ounce. Both had to do with "cell renewal" and pointed to "ultraviolet" damage that needed to be repaired by the two.

Night Repair told readers, "Use it tonight and wake up to better looking skin." This apparently rankled the competitor and the college professor.

However, Estée Lauder Night Repair ads sailed undisturbed until NAD's October 17, 1983 Case Report. Admitting that its investigation had been prompted by "independent challenges" from the competitor and the college professor, the advertising monitoring arm of the BBB said, "The competitor contributed a report of a preliminary biochemical study on Night Repair which it had commissioned ... [and] suggested that results indicated Night Repair had a negligible effect, if any, upon the cell repair process."

Although Lauder was able to satisfy some of NAD's inquiries, the group questioned whether the data supported claims of "dramatic first-night improvements" in skin condition. According to NAD, Lauder then "agreed to clarify that the improvements are most apparent with regular, nightly use."

On October 16, 1983, a day before NAD's announcement, Lauder's familiar double-page ad for Night Repair had appeared in the Sunday magazine section of *The New York Times*. Since ad space is reserved months ahead with the ads scattered to various publications, the unchanged Night Repair ad reappeared in the November 1983 issue of *Harper's Bazaar* and probably will continue to reappear until replaced by Estée Lauder's newest "scientific breakthrough" with its newest fractioned ounce at a new psychological price tag.

Unfortunately, no matter how much we would like to hold back the hands of time, no cream or potion has yet been found that will stop the clock of aging. Except for lines due to dryness, no wrinkle has been seen to disappear except through surgery. Still, it *is* possible to control the clock of aging, and it's up to us, individually, how or whether we slow it down—or speed it out of control.

Maintaining good health is the single best age retardant. What the entire body gets and does results in what you see and what is seen. Cosmetics can only help you groom and care for what you already have. Their power to change or camouflage is limited; but understanding their limitations and learning how to get the best and most out of the products you use can give you short- and long-term benefits.

If your finances are limited, don't be tempted into doing without necessities to spend more than a reasonable amount for cosmetics. Keep in mind that all cosmetic products, regardless of price, are subject to the same regulations or lack of regulations.

While a large company may have access to better facilities and, therefore, should be expected to have stricter company controls, famous-name brands, as well as others, have been involved in product seizures, recalls, and reprimands.

Particularly in makeup products such as powder, rouge, mascara, eye shadow, eyeliner, eyebrow pencil, and lipstick, many companies merely distribute the products that bear their names. A few large private-label manufacturers supply most of the makeup products for many of the companies whose names are known to consumers. These manufacturers also provide entire lines from creams to lip gloss for many other companies.

Often the same products appear under different names in the widest range of prices. A quick check through your medicine cabinet and dressing table will prove how many cosmetics, from hand lotion to deodorants to hair spray to creams and lipsticks, have the small-type telling words *"distributed by"* before the best-known as well as the lesser-known company names.

If you seriously care about how you look, begin with a physical checkup. If you're overweight, have your doctor provide you with a program of diet and exercise to get your body down to its proper weight and shape. Pass up the fad diets. The "yo-yo" syndrome of losing weight, regaining it, and losing it robs your skin of its elasticity.

Whatever shape your body is in, you can help it look

and stay better with good posture. How to stand, sit, and move will telegraph your age—true or not—to others. To prove it, walk down a busy street and, without looking at faces, try to guess the ages of those in front of you, those approaching you, and those passing you. The line of the spine will usually tell you more about the person than anything else.

To beat the clock, consciously keep your spine straight and your body in line *all the time,* not just when you know others are looking at you. It may be more comfortable to slump, but as you slump today, so may you be tomorrow.

It has been said that one is not responsible for one's appearance before twenty, but how one looks after forty is of one's own doing.

If you bake in the sun, without taking precautions, to flaunt a darker tan, it may be your undoing. Sunscreens are important, but so is discretion. Ultraviolet rays have been found to damage the skin, to cause wrinkling, and, in prolonged exposure, even to cause skin cancer. It is far better and more effective to use precaution than to attempt to undo damage with a cream or lotion, no matter what the price or the claims.

Teeth are seldom discussed in beauty "makeovers" and advice, and yet they are the most important facial structure. Regular visits to the dentist are a necessary insurance. Too many seem to be resorting to restorations rather than preservations.

When you are forced to resort to restoration, see that it is done promptly and well. All of us know people who are careful in all other aspects of their dress and appearance, yet neglect replacing missing back teeth. If a tooth must be lost, whether in front or back, it should be replaced as soon as possible, not only to protect other teeth, but also to protect your jaw and, consequently, the shape of your face.

Treasure every tooth you have by brushing after meals, and even after snacking, if you can. You don't have to use toothpaste each time. It's the brushing and flossing that count.

Telling, too, is John Galsworthy's observation that "One's eyes are what one is; one's mouth is what one becomes."

Tension, anger, bitterness, petulance—all shape the mouth. No amount of lipstick will hide a tight straight line or inverted crescent of a mouth. Consciously relaxing your mouth can help relieve the moment's tension. A sense of humor also helps. Better to have laugh lines than to scare dogs and little children.

Habitually frowning or creasing your brow also will endow you with more lines than will the calendar.

Motion-picture stars of past decades were said to have used pasties on their foreheads and smile lines to prevent permanent lines from forming. I don't know about the smile lines, but a few short pieces of transparent tape between your brows, in private, while you're sleeping, reading, or doing chores may keep you from unaware frowning and thereby hold off deeper lines.

If you wear glasses, have them checked periodically and change your frames with the times. Good-looking, becoming frames with subtly tinted lens can be a beauty treatment for the eyes. Also, if you need one, hearing aids are now so tiny and well designed that hair can easily make them invisible.

Once you've taken care of getting your health and body to their optimum, you're ready to gild the lily. Buy the best clothes you can afford. Try to stay with well-fitting quality classics. Pass up the faddish.

Put yourself in the hands of the best hairdresser you can find. If you don't have or know one, ask those whose hair-styling you admire for the name of their hairdresser. Keep your hairstyle simple and manageable. A good haircut is a prerequisite.

If you're happy with the natural color of your hair, treat it well by shampooing it frequently and conditioning it. There's no need to spend a great deal for shampoos and conditioners. Just get the simplest ones for your type of hair. The "additives" simply add to the cost and provide little else.

If you color your hair, stay away from the very dark or the very bright—as in black or red. If you've been a brunette, try going lighter. You'll find the lighter shades kinder to your face. If you have a great deal of gray or are almost white and would like color, try to get a shade that will blend in with your natural color rather than be in sharp contrast, so that you'll need fewer touch-ups as hair grows out. You may be able to make do with a rinse or a semipermanent color that gradually washes out with a number of shampoos and leaves no definite demarcation at the roots. Just be sure you don't succumb to rinses that turn you into a blue- or lavender-haired lady.

Finally, the less you subject your hair to dyes, permanents, straighteners, teasing, or blow-drying, the better. Use a shampoo and conditioner for color-treated hair. Keep brushing to a minimum, and use a pomade to give it a sheen.

Your allover skin needs more care as you grow older. If you're in the sun, even if you're not sunbathing, a sunscreen is a must.

To keep your skin soft, bath oil in your bath helps, along with a water softener if your water is hard. A hand and body lotion is one of the most useful cosmetic staples. Smooth the lotion over your entire body while your skin is still damp after your bath and don't forget your feet, including the soles.

At night, take your makeup off with a light cleansing cream or plain mineral oil. Rinse with warm water and go over your face with a soft washcloth. Then wash your face with a mild or superfatted soap. If washing your face with soap leaves it too dry, try using a wash-off cream or cleanser. Either way, rinse your face well with a number of rinsings, avoiding very hot or very cold water. Follow up with a cream to moisturize. A heavier, richer cream could be used on your throat and around your eyes. If you find a cream irritating to your eyes, use plain petroleum jelly.

To keep the skin on your hands smooth and supple, use a hand cream or lotion on your hands after washing, whenever possible. An easy way to remember is to leave a small pump bottle of hand lotion on each sink.

In the morning, rinse your face well and go over it with a damp washcloth before you put on a light cream or lotion as a foundation for your makeup. If you don't find it too drying, you could go over your face, after rinsing, with a cotton dampened with a very mild freshener or a few drops of alcohol mixed with water, then rinse again, before smoothing on a cream or lotion.

Before you even think about making up, be sure you have a strong magnifying mirror in the brightest light possible and keep your glasses handy if you wear them. Too many older women look as though they've made up in the dark.

If your skin is good, with good color, all you'll probably need is a moisturizer. As you get older, the less makeup you wear, the better and younger you'll look. If you need some color, you can use a blusher, which should be blended so that it looks like a faint blush with no visible edges.

Although the dry brush-on blushers have become popular, these are more successfully used over powder. When face powder is not worn, my preference is a cream rouge blended with foundation, as I was shown by one of Elizabeth Arden's makeup instructors a number of years ago.

Dab a dot of cream rouge on the edge of your palm. Add a drop of liquid foundation and blend the two together to tone down the rouge into a more believable flesh tone. The thinner consistency will help the color go on more easily and make it easier to blend it into naturalness. This works as well if you need and wear a colored foundation.

If you wear a colored foundation, be sure it blends with your skin color and keep it a light film. Some makeup artists thin the foundation by mixing it with a little water. You could do the same by mixing just enough foundation with water or a moisturizing lotion in your palm before applying it. If necessary, dust a light film of colorless powder to set your makeup. Also, if necessary, you can add a flick of brush-on blusher. Then, smooth it all with a soft makeup sponge or with your hands so there's no powdery film. Or you can pat your face with a slightly damp sponge, as Linda Evans' favorite makeup artist, Armando Cosio, does.

Steer clear of any heavy or obvious makeup. It doesn't cover; it only makes whatever lines or wrinkles you may have more noticeable.

Your eyes should be softly and subtly shadowed with a light tracing of neutral shadow—a soft taupe, gray, or smoky brown. Shadow should look like a natural shadow and not a bright green or blue eyeshade.

If you use an eyeliner, try using a taupe, dark gray, or similar shade rather than black, and use it on just the outside half or three-quarters of your eyes. This will give extension to your eyes rather than closing them up. Soften the line by smudging it with your finger or a sponge-tipped swab and then clean up the rough edges with a cotton swab.

Use mascara on your upper lashes only. If you wear glasses, put them on, and clean up the misses with a cotton swab dampened with water or lotion, depending on the mas-

cara. Usually, your eyebrows should be left as they are, except
for tweezing any stray hairs. Just brush the brows into place
with the tiniest trace of petroleum jelly, if necessary.

When you use makeup, keep it light and natural. Be
sure to extend your foundation and powder to your neck and
blend it so that there is no line of demarcation. The effect
should be of a natural blooming and not one of being "made
up."

Looking well and being well groomed, *at any age,* takes
more time and work than it does dollars. It may take a little
longer and a little more work with each birthday, but the results should be worth it.

All of us grow older. The key word is *grow.* As we grow
older, we hope we also grow in character and grow wiser, more
tolerant, and into more interesting individuals. We should be
able to laugh at ourselves, be more comfortable with ourselves,
and discover that we like ourselves pretty well. We also realize
that though we're growing older, we'll never be old.

Or as Oliver Wendell Holmes said on the seventieth
birthday of Julia Ward Howe, "To be seventy years young is
sometimes far more cheerful and hopeful than to be forty years
old."

QUESTIONS AND ANSWERS

**How successful are the bleaching creams that are supposed to
fade age or liver spots?**

During a radio interview, Princess Marcella Borghese,
whose name appears on one of the higher-priced Revlon lines,
said her most difficult problem was trying to get rid of the
brown spots that appear with age.

If the accumulated pigment is flat, and you can pinpoint the cream, you might be able to lighten it in time. However, you'll probably be lightening the skin around it as well and may wind up with a halo that's lighter than the surrounding skin. If the pigmented spot is raised, the cream will do little if anything to correct the problem.

What about facial exercises? Will they help avoid wrinkles as claimed?

According to Dr. Behrman and other dermatologists, facial exercises can do more harm than good. As Dr. Behrman pointed out, our faces are constantly in motion when we eat, speak, drink, smile, laugh, and otherwise exercise our faces in the normal routine of living; and it's precisely because of repeated motion that lines are formed.

Are facials recommended?

Not if they involve manipulating the skin, using steam, or very hot or cold applications. The older skin should be treated gently without being stretched, manipulated, or subjected to extremes in temperature.

In the winter, my skin, especially on my legs, becomes so dry it looks as though it's almost cracking. What can be done to help relieve this condition?

Cold weather has a way of drying and chapping skin, and, often, dry heat within our homes compounds the damage. Try getting more moisture in your home—the old practice of a pan of water on the radiator still works—and use an inexpensive hand and body lotion all over your body after each bath or shower. For your legs, try an inexpensive cream, oil, or petroleum jelly, rubbed in so it's no longer greasy. Boots also help battle the elements outdoors during the winter.

I am in my sixties and find that the makeup I've been using looks heavier than I like even though I try to use it sparingly.

I'm now using a moisturizer, foundation, rouge, powder, lipstick, eye shadow, eyebrow pencil and liner, and mascara.

Without knowing the shades of makeup you're using and your coloring, it's difficult to recommend a detailed plan for improvement. However, the biggest mistake some older women make is to use too much makeup in too glaring or dark colors.

Using a moisturizer, foundation, and powder may be too much and may tend to emphasize lines and wrinkles. If you have a good skin tone, try using just a moisturizer with a light dusting of powder and then a powdered blusher. If you feel you must use a foundation, use a light moisturizing lotion and a thin fluid foundation without powder for a moist look. The key is to keep the film *thin*. Blend in a pastel cream rouge. Also, try using a dampened sponge to set your makeup. Or you might try a trick that's taught at a modeling school. The models are taught to put on their makeup and then blend it with a dry sponge until most of the makeup is off and just a nice natural glow is left.

As for the rest of your makeup, stay away from bright blue, green, or violet eye shadow. Use a faint shadow in taupe shades that look like real shadow. Your lipstick should be no darker than a medium shade; avoid pearlized or muddy tones. Use everything even more sparingly than, apparently, you have been. You probably don't need to pencil your eyebrows; just smooth them with a brush . . . and, please, no heavy eyeliners.

— 21 —
Saving Face and Saving Money

Since curiosity and temptation are always with
us, you alone must decide whether a product is
worth its price to you.
—Toni Stabile

If ever you have questioned whether label prestige warranted the prestigious price being charged for a cosmetic that was kin to another with a proletarian label, a discovery by the FDA in the 1960s may hold the answer to your question.

It was a time when many women were complaining of problems with irritated eyes and eyelids. Before I knew the reason, I'd noticed an attractive model who had come into a New York beauty salon to have her hair done. She was wearing dark glasses, which she reluctantly took off so that the hairdresser could begin the shampoo. Behind the glasses, her eyelids were red and swollen. She had never been allergic to anything, she told the hairdresser, but she had been using this new eyeliner ...

In the same building, I kept an appointment with a

magazine editor. She complained that her eyes itched and smarted, and added that she'd never been allergic to anything—but maybe she wasn't getting enough sleep . . .

In the Washington office of FDA's Division of Color and Cosmetics, a letter arrived describing a reaction similar to that suffered by the model. The writer of the letter claimed that her eyelids had swollen after she had used an eyeliner pencil, and named the brand and shade she had used. The FDA tested the pencil and was surprised to find that it contained coal-tar color forbidden for use around the eyes since 1938, when Lash Lure's shocking blinding and death prompted the first cosmetic legislation.

"Then," an FDA spokesman told me, "we wondered what would happen if we tested some other pencils. We tested and darned if they didn't have coal-tar colors—and then others . . ."

FDA soon found that a number of shades in practically every brand tested had coal-tar dye. At a time when fashion decreed eye makeup to be as essential as lipstick, it suddenly became difficult to find eyeliners on the counters as the FDA seized almost one million pencils containing the illegal dye, and the manufacturers and distributors recalled several million more.

For alert consumers, the eye-pencil seizures held a peculiar twist in customer industry revelation. While famous name companies were selling their pencils for $1.50 and more, other companies were filling variety-store counters with twenty-nine-cent pencils.

According to the FDA: "We found that this one fellow in Tennessee, who was supplying the crayon cores used in almost all the pencils, was putting coal-tar color in them."

The "fellow in Tennessee" was Jensen's, Inc., in Shelbyville, producer of 115,000 eye pencils a week. Jensen's was reported as having told a *New York Times* reporter that the banned colors had been on the market for nine years before being picked up by the FDA. According to FDA and TGA (now CTFA) sources, Jensen's pleaded ignorance of the law.

Replying to this, the agency spokesman said, "Jensen's should have known. Their customers also should have been testing the color material as part of quality control which is a necessary part of any pretesting program."

Among the labels on pencils with the illegal cores listed by the FDA were: Avon, Marian Bialac, Hazel Bishop, Cosmetically Yours, Debutante, Max Factor, Ann Harper, Maybelline, Elizabeth Post, Revlon, Helena Rubinstein, and Smartee, which also had a liquid eyeliner containing coal-tar color.

Some of the companies behind the labels claimed that they had spot-checked the eye makeup from time to time, but since the coal-tar colors were not present in all shades, the offenders had been missed. Other companies claimed that Jensen's had changed the formula since their last check. Then, too, they said they'd relied on a supplier guarantee that the products did not contain coal-tar dyes.

At the time, I wrote to Jensen's asking for the reason for the slip-up on a regulation in effect since 1938—a regulation that was well known to the cosmetic industry. I received no reply. Also unanswered were questions about steps taken to correct the infringement and its recurrence, and whether any injuries or reactions from the coal-tar colors had been reported.

Other questions such as "Was any action other than the seizures taken against Jensen's by the FDA or others?" were partly answered by FDA, which said it had taken no further action, and "Have you lost any customers because of the incident?" by the TGA, which said no.

The Merck Index, prepared for industry reference, had

this caution about coal tar: "Continuous contact with the skin for long periods may result in dermatitis and skin cancer."

Although a million pencils were seized and destroyed and several million more recalled (after FDA caught up with the violation), there is no indication that anything was done about the pencils already sold to the public. No warning notice appeared. No ad offered the unwary consumer a new pencil for the forbidden one.

At the time of the FDA pickup operation, Revlon was running stunningly colored ads that included the line: "Revlon's enticing range of 65 eye shades can do no wrong, day or night!"

Meanwhile, the suffering model and editor decided they'd better throw away their eyeliners, both brands later picked up by FDA as offenders. Neither reported her reaction. Both discarded their $1.50 pencils and bought other brands for $1.50. Both took exactly the same risk they'd taken before. The labels were different, but the pencils were the same. But, then, how could they have known about "this one fellow in Tennessee"?

In the 1980s, eyeliner pencils are tagged with prices that have tripled and quadrupled since the 1960s. Big-name companies with big advertising budgets are charging $6.50 per pencil. But, just as in the sixties, when pencils could be had in a range of prices, some one-fifth the price of others, so, too, can they be had in the eighties. In fact, private label companies will supply pencils with your name on them if you want to get into the cosmetic business. One pencil will cost you thirty cents. If you order more than 720 pencils, you can get them for twenty cents. And it's very possible that you'll be getting the same pencil that may be wearing a popular label and a $6.50 price tag.

The range of prices can be much more than one to five

or even one to ten times for basically the same cosmetic. According to the merchandiser of one of the country's largest stores, the only difference between the dollar cream and the $20 cream was packaging (although it was in a plain jar), advertising, *and psychological pricing.*

It's up to you whether you feel it's worth the price of the hope that Steve Mayham, the industry spokesman, said the cosmetic industry was selling. If the price seems unreasonable to you, it probably is. Most of us have accepted aspirin under generic brands because we've been convinced that aspirin is aspirin under any label. Maybe it's time to think generically about the cosmetics we use.

First, we must get over the idea that the most advertised cosmetics are the most desirable. When a company spends eight to twenty million dollars to launch a new cosmetic, it is betting that it can persuade you into picking up the tab by paying more than the product would otherwise cost.

When you consider that you were sold by last year's promotion by the same company that promised its last year's product would make you instantly beautiful and forever young, why then aren't those promises valid for that product this year? Besides, didn't you pay that unreasonable price for that little miracle-worker and then find it did no more for you than the old stuff you'd been using that cost a tenth of the price for a larger size? In fact, the fancy cream with the fancy price may have made your face break out.

The cosmetic industry *thrives* on change. Most consumers do not thrive on change. Apart from depleting the purse, changing from cosmetic to cosmetic can take its toll in sensitization, allergic reactions, and other adverse reactions. When you use a cosmetic, you're using it on living tissue— *yours.* It is not a new scouring powder being tried on your sink.

Think twice before you sit down to have a demonstrator make up your face with a line of products and give you a chart with a list of all the cosmetics you should buy to make you irresistible. Take a look at the demonstrator and the person behind the counter. Really look and see if those products have created a miracle, taking into account the pesky nature of genes. Then look and see how sanitary those cosmetics are while they are being smeared on one and all. Your skin and body may be able to cope with its own bacteria, but are they able to cope with invading troupes of foreign bacteria?

I'm constantly amazed at the open "samplers" that are allowed in department and specialty stores. Week after week, uncovered displays of lip gloss, eye shadow, cream rouge, and other makeup are on countertops to be "sampled." Amid the pretension of glamour, no one, including the health authorities, seems to notice that the dust- and dirt-gritted pots are potential harbors of unfriendly bacteria to be carried away by those who accept the invitation to sample.

I have watched demonstrators make up person after person, dipping into the same makeup jars and tubes. Although consumers are told not to use other people's mascaras, I observed no new tubes of mascara being opened for each demonstratee, no fresh lipstick, or eye shadow. The makeup brushes were dipped into an apparently sanitizing solution that became cloudy and unappealing as the sessions went on. The brushes, however, were not dipped and sanitized each time they were dipped into the demonstrator's supplies. I also noticed that some of the dry brushes which were used to blend powder and blushers were not sanitized at all. Is it any wonder that some women have complained of getting blemishes, rashes, or other adverse reactions after a "makeup lesson"?

Cosmetics should be fun, but their use should be tempered by common sense. The cosmetic industry, however, has bent the rules in Washington by playing the "risk assessment" game, which is supposed to pit the risks against benefits.

The fallacy in the game is that cosmetics are neither

food, which is necessary to sustain life, nor drugs, which are meant to save life, repair, or restore health—in which case, risk to benefit becomes a valid evaluation. Without being life-sustaining or life-saving, cosmetics are intended only to make life more pleasant by allowing us to look and smell a little better. Why, then, should the consumer be forced to take a risk while the cosmetic companies reap the benefits?

If the cosmetic companies want to use the counter samplings and demonstrations to sell their products, why not package the samplings in individual sample packets? There are companies that specialize in individual packets, tubes, and vials. It may mean some added expense, but the cost is in pennies, and the cosmetics that are being sold are profitable enough so that the pennies would be lost in their calculations. One young woman with a beginning job was talked into buying $140 worth of cosmetics in one session at one counter. Most of the products were worthless to her as well as unnecessary.

In the interest of making you a winner instead of a loser in the cosmetics game, here are some rules for playing with the least financial risk. If your risk is primarily in giving a sensitive skin more trouble than it can take, I suggest you indulge your curiosity as little as possible and stay with whatever you know agrees with your skin.

1. Look in newspapers, magazines, and stores for sample and trial offers of products that interest you.

2. Take advantage of package deals that have attached samples that you can try, and then return the regular-size package if the sample doesn't please you.

3. Take advantage of products sold with a guarantee of satisfaction and *return* them if they don't satisfy. (Actually, the guarantee of satisfaction is implicit in most established products.)

4. Return products that produce the wrong reaction— that cause any irritation, itching, swelling, or other unpleasant-

ness involving any part of the body. Be alert for any discomfort to eyes and nails and, while using hairsprays, coughing or any other difficulty in breathing. Avoid deodorants or antiperspirants in spray forms.

5. Return products that don't live up to their label or advertising claims. If they don't, they're in violation of FDA or FTC regulations.

6. If you encounter unreasonable resistance from salespeople, ask to see the manager. If you're not satisfied at the departmental level, write to a store executive or write directly to the cosmetic company.

7. Try one product at a time in its smallest size. If it proves to be the right one for you, watch for periodic sales. Most companies or stores have half-price or special sales at various intervals so you can stock up and cut the cost of cosmetics. However, don't buy more than you can use in a reasonable time. Without dates to show the recommended product life, cosmetics should be looked upon as perishables even though you may find supposedly "recalled" cosmetics on some shelves three or more years after the announced recall.

8. If you still find yourself spending more than you'd like on cosmetics, check the private-label brands (the store's own brands) of popular-price, variety, drug, or discount stores. Compare contents and prices and try the one that gives you most for the least cost. Since all cosmetics are subject to the same government standards and regulations, such as they are, the one that agrees with your skin and body at the lowest cost is the one for you. Don't be misled by others' raves about other products. What may be great for another may be less than great for you.

9. Learn to resist being sold "sets" of cosmetics on the basis of a loaded analysis for a "routine" that's supposed to make you a raving beauty by next week or because they "go to-

gether." Go slowly, buy only what you need, and resist being sold the large economy size until you know you're suited. Once you know you're right for each other, buy it and *use* it.

10. Keep in mind that the fewer beauty items you use to keep yourself well groomed and your skin clean and supple, the less likely you are to have a collection of dead enthusiasm bought with live money.

QUESTIONS AND ANSWERS

Does a "new look" require a whole set of new makeup? I'd like to update my appearance and I'm told I must buy several new products, which can be very expensive.

Unless there has been a marked change in the color of your hair or skin, there's no need for a whole set of new and expensive makeup. Try one product at a time and spend some time with a mirror in different lights. Start with a new lipstick, which needn't be expensive if you concentrate on color instead of a name label. Once you find the right shade for you, you may find that the rest of your makeup is still right. Just as important as the right shades is the way you use your makeup for your particular features as well as for the occasion and your way of life.

I'd like to use an eyeliner to give better definition to my eyes, but I find the eyeliners rather too hard to draw a soft line easily.

There are softer eyeliners, some of which are designated as "kohl." Before applying the liners, some makeup artists soften the tips by dipping them into lotion or cream. Another warms the pencil between the palms of his hands. I prefer running warm water over the point of the liner before using it. Whatever you choose, just be sure that the eyeliner around your eyes is muted and not a hard dark line. It should be a mere hint of shadow and should appear as though it is the natural rim of your eyelashes.

I have difficulty finding the right shade of lipstick. I have a whole bunch of lipsticks that looked right in the store and wrong when I got home and put them on. How can I get the right shade?

Maybe you can get the right shade without buying still another lipstick. Use the ones you have to mix the colors on your lips until you get the shade you want. Usually you can get the right shade by using two lipsticks, one shade applied over the other. Blot after the first application so you don't have a build-up. If you like, you can also blot after the second application.

Another way of arriving at the right shade is to use the lipstick that's closest to what you want and top it with a tinted lip gloss in a shade that brings the lipstick into the color you want.

I have tried the pump sprays and the aerosols in hairsprays. I realize that you get more product for your money in the pump sprays, but I find that I can get a finer mist with the aerosols. Still, I don't like breathing in that spray.

The pump-spray people probably are working toward producing finer sprays. In the interest of your hair, however, I suggest that any hairspray be used sparingly and only when you find it to be absolutely necessary.

When using hairspray, or any other sprays, directly on yourself, use them defensively by spraying in an open room instead of in a closed bathroom, then leave the room so that you don't inhale the spray.

I've been using a well-known brand of petroleum jelly as a lubricant and moisturizer for my skin, but in recent years, I find

**the price has been raised to the point that it costs almost as
much as some creams.**

You probably can blame the price rise on increased advertising for the product as well as inflation, but petroleum jelly is petroleum jelly, and you can find respectable private-label brands at a fraction of the one that's heavily advertised. In fact, at a recent sale in a national variety store, I was able to buy a one-pound jar of petroleum jelly for ninety-nine cents . . . a *small* fraction of the price of the advertised brand. The only difference I could distinguish between the two was the label.

— 22 —
Are We Ready for "Risk Assessment"?

The men who control the industry are talking to
each other when they should take some time to
talk to the consumers.
—Toni Stabile

The late Stephen L. Mayham, who was the TGA-CTFA spokesman and the voice of the cosmetic industry for twenty-five years, said it best. "What we sell in cosmetics," he said, "is hope."

Consumers have responded by buying hope at the rate of approximately $12.5 billion a year, excluding the products and services bought in beauty and barber shops.

The recent "risk-assessment" policy on questioned color additives proposed by The Cosmetic, Toiletry and Fragrance Association, which represents the cosmetic industry, and espoused by the Food and Drug Administration, which is supposed to protect consumers, amounts to a thumbing of collective noses at the taxpaying consumers who pay to keep both operations afloat.

During an interview with CTFA President Ed Kavanaugh, I suggested that those responsible for what we find in the market are out of phase with the actual buyer. So many of the executives and top personnel, including those of the FDA, the cosmetic industry, and the CTFA, are so busy running around talking to each other that they don't have contact with the average person who buys and uses the products.

"Well," Mr. Kavanaugh replied, "CTFA doesn't get into any of the marketing part."

I reminded him that *that* was the end result. "That's why you're there," I told him.

Speaking for the CTFA, its president claimed: "We're here to provide a different service or function to our members. What the board of directors, in effect, said to CTFA is to work in the regulatory, legislative arena, legal arena, scientific arena, to help show the safety of these products. But when it comes to marketing what the consumer wants, the companies are doing that on their own. And that's a very competitive world out there."

I agreed, but pointed out that, in the final analysis, even the CTFA would not be funded if it were not funded by the cosmetic industry, and if, in turn, the cosmetic industry were not being funded by the consumers. I also reminded him of my observation while I was testifying during the Senate hearings on the Eagleton cosmetic safety bill after the cadre of CTFAers complained that any change in regulation would cost consumers an inordinate amount for additional labeling. (Other testimony established the amount as half a cent.)

Amid all the threatening by industry representatives that the consumer would be soaked heavily for any change in the status quo and all the professed concern about the consumer's purse being depleted by labeling costs, I wondered about the money that had been spent on unsuccessful cosmetic promotions that had cost millions instead of pennies.

"Was not the consumer soaked for it anyway?" I asked, adding, "And, also, I might say that the consumer is paying for both sides of this [witness] table. One of the gentlemen here is staying at the Madison [one of D.C.'s most expensive hotels]. Who is picking up that tab? We are going to pay for it."

Senator Eagleton: "Half is picked up by the Internal Revenue Service and half by the consumer."

        I: "And who keeps the Internal Revenue Service going?"

Senator Eagleton: "Right."

Yet, with the consumer-taxpayer footing the bills for all concerned, the consumer-taxpayer has little to do with what is found in the marketplace. The cosmetic industry plays its game of hits and misses, and the consumers pay for the industry's misses with the prices tagged on new products and with the prices raised on existing products.

In Washington, the legislators and regulators get their paychecks and perks regardless of their actions or inactions, and the taxpayers pay for the inactions as well as for the actions that often act against them.

When it comes to assessing risks, the risks are assessed against the consumers who are expected and encouraged to pay for taking the risks ... like obediently trusting human guinea pigs.

The cosmetic industry has planned the biggest promotional blitz in its history in an effort to promote its risk-to-benefit theory—or how to play the cosmetic game of Russian roulette for fun and profit. No matter how slickly the promotion is packaged, consumers will still be taking whatever the risks may be while the industry reaps the benefits.

In contrast to the highly paid and skilled trade association with its political action committees intended to affect legislation and regulation, it seems that we, the paying patsies, are lonely voices at the bottom of the barrel, unheard and unheeded.

My explorations in the field of cosmetics have brought me into contact not only with members of the industry, the regulatory and legislative branches of government, but, most importantly, with literally thousands of consumers. Increasingly, I have found an inverted ratio of concern between what might be termed "them" and "us."

As consumers become more aware and desirous of safety, purity, and dependability in the products they use in and on their bodies and in the environment, those responsible for the safety, purity, and dependability of those products seemingly have become more determined to practice laissez-faire and more active in attempting to warp or abolish the meager consumer safeguards that were won after decades of excruciating effort. The determined activity to return to the dark ages of consumer-beware-and-be-damned found its ally in the recent years of executive guillotining orders.

Cosmetics must be recognized for what they are. They are intended to make life more pleasant, more attractive, and more comfortable. They are neither life-sustaining nor life-saving. Unlike drugs, which are selectively used and where a benefit may outweigh a risk, there is no justification for risk in cosmetics other than the possibility of an allergic reaction in some individuals.

As for color additives, it seems irrational to spend years and millions of dollars identifying a carcinogen only to then attempt to make the carcinogen palatable by implying that consumers should gamble on the odds just to have a redder fake strawberry icing or another imperceptibly different shade of lipstick. In the blackest comedy being played in Washington, the industry and the FDA have joined in giving consumer odds in a cancer lottery, apparently ignoring the unavoidable odds already in place for consumers who, if asked, might prefer not to take one more unnecessary gamble.

Even a cursory examination of the odds being presented exposes the fallacy of attempting to cite odds on what cannot be considered to be a sound, factual basis. The entire policy of risk assessment can be no more than a "guestimate," since there is no human experience on which to base the projection. The industry cannot produce the results of a controlled study of human beings who have been exposed only to the suspected color additive over the two or three decades it may require for a cancer to appear.

The risk assessments have come from industry-conducted tests on animals with statistics compiled and interpreted by industry-paid statisticians. On the other hand, to my knowledge, there has yet to be anyone who can determine how much of a carcinogen or how many carcinogens it takes to trigger a cancer, or to accelerate an existing cancer in any one person, or at which age and condition of health and with which degree of susceptibility. Nothing has been said of the possibility of interaction between carcinogens among human beings who now are being equated with the very animals that were rejected as barometers by the cosmetic industry when it found it to be convenient to do so.

To what end should we welcome the industry's risk assessments when we're told to weigh the risks to the benefits? Where are the benefits to the consumers who are being handed the risks? Obviously the benefits have seesawed to the seat of the industry. What possible benefit could it be to a consumer to have Revlon boast that it has hundreds of shades of lipstick, and for a supplier to offer more hundreds of shades of eye shadow?

Having spent a great deal of time with consumers, I have found the general opinion among them is that they can do

244 EVERYTHING YOU WANT TO KNOW ABOUT COSMETICS

nicely without 160 shades of any cosmetic if it means taking risks. In fact, many of them pointed out that they'd be satisfied with much fewer, kept in place, so that when they went back to the store for a lipstick they could find it available. In other words, throw out the questionable colors and get on with providing safe, dependable cosmetics in shades that will not disappear with next season's promotion.

Thus far, the consumer's only bulwark against cancer-causing additives has been the Delaney Amendment to the Food, Drug, and Cosmetic Act which, since 1958, has barred the use of any additive shown to cause cancer in man or animal. Although cosmetics were included in the bill, the usual pressure prevailed, and as had happened with past bills, cosmetics were dropped before the amendment became law. Color additives, however, remained, since they affected food and drugs as well as cosmetics. The loudest cries, reactions, and evasive actions have come from the cosmetic industry.

Now that Congressman James J. Delaney has retired, various factions are intent on cannibalizing the amendment. Bills have been introduced to provide the industry with the loopholes they seek. In the wings, political action committees go over the lists of the "right" legislators, and the industry public-relation machines are busy with their campaigns to "re-educate" the public on the nirvana of "risk assessment." As the Delaney Amendment stands, it now has no loopholes—*and that seems to please no one but the consumers.*

QUESTIONS AND ANSWERS

Why can't the cosmetic industry be satisfied with the colors that have been approved and forget the questionable ones?
I have been asking the same question for years. The

only explanation that has been given is that the companies want them, and what the industry wants, the industry usually gets.

After twenty-three years, shouldn't the questions of color safety have been resolved?

One would think so, yet in November 1983, an acting FDA commissioner was reported as having complimented the CTFA, acting for the cosmetic industry, as having only ten colors left to be resolved. In the meantime, the cosmetic industry has had a free ride on questionably safe colors that have been in limbo on the provisional list for twenty-three years.

Why has "risk assessment" suddenly become the clarion call?

No one is saying, but conjecture has it that the climate in Washington is right for the industry's regaining any measures it may have lost to consumers in the past. The industry-stroking climate also may be the reason for the cosmetic industry being suddenly desirous of getting all the remaining provisional colors permanently listed quickly.

Fortunately for the industry, and unfortunately for consumers, the most questionable colors remain on the provisional list. Tests on some of these colors have shown them to have carcinogens in their constituents, which the FDA has approved. Others now are being shown to have carcinogens in the actual color additives, which are forbidden by the Delaney Amendment. Apparently, that is the reason the CTFA has sought allies among some of the legislators to introduce legislation that will bore convenient holes in the Delaney Amendment for the cosmetic industry to slide through.

What can we do to avoid having "risk assessments" we'd rather not have in our cosmetic or food colors?

Complain, complain, complain ... by writing to your senator and congressman ... writing to the FDA commissioner and the Secretary of Health and Human Services; to The Cosmetic, Toiletry and Fragrance Association in Washington, D.C.; and to the companies responsible for the cosmetics you buy and use. If you're in personal touch with your legislators, let them know how you feel about any bills that threaten to weaken the Delaney Amendment. You may not have the dollars of a political action committee, but you do have your vote—and it's your vote that counts in keeping or ousting a legislator in Washington.

— 23 —
The Industry

They should admit that there are two parts to the
industry and that one part is not performing the
way it should.
—Donald A. Davis, Editor,
Drug & Cosmetic Industry

A peculiar situation exists in the American cosmetic industry. The industry has evolved into the big business it is today only within the last half-century. Even the industry associations have records only as far back as the 1930s.

Although cosmetics have been compounded and used almost as long as men and women have existed, not until the turn of this century, when less than a handful of women concocted creams and potions in their kitchens, bathtubs, and garages, were cosmetics dignified as "manufactured" products and distributed to ever widening circles of consumers.

In less than sixty years, the American cosmetic industry has evolved from a bathtub-and-garage operation to an international big business, blanketing the world with seductive advertising and charted on every stock exchange.

Dismissed by Congress as unimportant in 1906, the sketchy cosmetics used by a minority at the turn of the century were even then on their way to becoming as staple as salt and aspirin to the majority. The American passion for personal enhancement and sexual attractiveness, already being exploited by medicine men and unbridled advertising, encouraged the development of a continuing variety of products that ranged from shampoo and toothpaste to deodorants and foot powder. Hope-filled names such as "Beautifying Wash" and "Virginal Milk" vied with "slimming creams" in all-promising ads.

By the 1930s, the unbridled industry had erupted to anything-goes with no holds barred. With no controls and no checks, anything and everything could be thrown into a package, advertised any way it pleased the advertiser, and the easy profits reaped even though there might be victims along the way. Eventually, the reports of death and maimings from "beauty" products became too frequent and horrendous to be ignored.

One depilatory, Kormelu, contained thallium acetate, a rat poison, and sold for years at $10 a jar even after it had been proved to have caused baldness, pain, and paralysis. Comparatively little publicity was given to the injuries as the depilatory continued to be advertised as "entirely safe for face, arms, and legs."

In an attempt to move Congress into action, a display of fraudulent and/or harmful products was assembled in the FDA chief inspector's office, which was christened "The Chamber of Horrors" by reporters. After Congress and pressure groups jousted for five years, the Food, Drug, and Cosmetic Act was passed in 1938. That, coupled with the same-year passage of the Wheeler-Lee Amendment to the Federal Trade Commission Act, extending the commission's powers over false and misleading advertising to include protection for the consumers as well as for competitors, resulted in a vigorous sweep of offenders by the FDA and FTC.

Still, the cosmetic industry remained uniquely free of meaningful controls, and it took another thirty-nine years before the FDA forced cosmetic companies to list the ingredients. Even with the loopholes that allow small amounts of ingredients, fragrances, and trade secrets to escape labeling, ingredient labeling is responsible for prompting The Cosmetic, Toiletry and Fragrance Association into attempting to lead its members into the twentieth century.

However, with the relaxed surveillance of the cosmetic industry by the FDA and the somnolence of the FTC, a dark side of the cosmetic industry has reverted to a number of bathtub-and-garage operations throughout the country with advertising from even prestigious CTFA members that is reminiscent of medicine-men days.

On the one hand, there is what Don Davis calls "the establishment," which includes the members of CTFA and the major cosmetic companies. When the CTFA or the major companies speak as the voice of the industry, they speak only for that segment and cannot claim to speak for the entire cosmetic industry.

On the other hand, there are numerous companies that are not part of the establishment. Many may not have heard of the CTFA or regulations. Most are not registered and are unknown to the FDA and, therefore, escape inspections.

A tour of local stores will convince anyone that the shelved cosmetic products of major companies with familiar names share the space with an almost equal number of products with unfamiliar names from unrecognized companies. As CTFA Ed Kavanaugh said, "There's an awful lot of product out there."

Some of the unrecognized companies may be following

the best manufacturing procedures and may be producing excellent, dependable, and pristine products. Others, however, may be of the bathtub-and-garage school, producing contaminated and questionable products that are likely to sail past all checks until and unless an adversely affected consumer brings the product to someone's attention.

Don Davis' suggestion that the CTFA recognize those on the other side of the tracks and try to bring them into the twentieth century by asking Congress to pass legislation to make the voluntary program of company registration, formula disclosure, and adverse reaction reporting mandatory.

When told that it was more than unlikely that the CTFA or the establishment would ask for *any* legislation, Mr. Davis replied, "*That's the point!* They won't, because of their basic contention that the industry is all pristine white. And you don't have an industry that's like that. You have a profoundly divided industry that consists of some companies that are ethical and some companies that are so nonethical, it's incredible.

"If, at least, they got the ethical industry, or if they got all the CTFA members to conform to even the voluntary program, they'd be that much ahead."

Simple registration of the companies with the FDA would be a step in the right direction. If the states of Florida could mandate registration, why should the nation be so far behind?

According to Mr. Davis, if the establishment and the CTFA, which represents it, are willing to make the admission that there are others practicing outside the establishment, and work from there, the entire industry would change for the better.

"It will have to," he emphasized. "It doesn't have to be on a trade association level. The outsiders will either have to toe the line or be cited by the FDA every time it comes through on an inspection if only that voluntary program were converted to a mandatory status. Just that alone would help the FDA do a whole lot more.

"That's just the first step. I'm not saying it should be the last. But the cosmetic establishment is unwilling to take the first step.

"Now you have the industry defending a whole bunch of pirates and bathtub operators out there. What should be done, instead, is to ease those pirates and operators out of the industry, or at least bring them in line with the rest of the cosmetic establishment. Failing that, they must be forced into a profile where the FDA could take a shot at them. Give the FDA more guns, in other words. Those people then would either be put out of business or made to conform to basic cleanliness or whatever standards are necessary for good manufacturing practice. Then a substantial part of the industry would be nearly in compliance now."

With the laissez-faire attitude prevalent in the 1980s among the industry representatives, regulators, and legislators, who have taken their cue from the administration, we have the peculiar situation of a bathtub operation of the pre-1930s going on at the same time that we have the CTFA dragging its companies into the twentieth century.

As Don Davis put it: "You have these two different divisions in the industry, led by the more ethical end of the business, which has some very good companies who do very good work, being tarnished by the image of these other people.

"That's really the problem in the industry, and it's something you can't break down because the industry establishment isn't willing to admit that those other people exist."

CTFA's voice of the establishment, Ed Kavanaugh, reiterated that CTFA had testified at Senate hearings on the

Eagleton Cosmetic Safety Act of 1974, chaired by Senator Edward A. Kennedy, and, again, in 1975, that it had no objection to making the voluntary program mandatory in the form it was in. However, CTFA's Chairman of the Board J. Richard Edmondson, vice-president of Bristol-Myers, also testified that the purpose of his statement was "to indicate that any new legislation is unwise and unnecessary."

It has been a firm policy of the CTFA, and the TGA before it, to oppose vigorously any legislation of any kind that touches the cosmetic industry. They have been successful in knocking out cosmetics from every bill before it could become law, before and after the weak-sister addition of cosmetics to the Food, Drug, and Cosmetic Act in 1938. The CTFA moved to the steps of Congress in Washington, D.C., from New York City expressly to monitor government action and to abort any measures that might wind up as regulation or legislation.

What isn't mentioned is that to make the voluntary program mandatory *requires new legislation*, which the CTFA and the cosmetic industry opposed. To repeat the offer is sweetly safe.

It may be well to note that the CTFA offered the voluntary program during the 1970s when there were a number of bills in the House and Senate that would have mandated premarket testing as well as stricter controls on cosmetics. Consumers and consumer advocates had been alerted to the problems that had been overlooked in cosmetics, and Professor Joseph A. Page had begun a postgraduate seminar on Lawyering in the Public Interest, prompted by my first book, *Cosmetics: Trick or Treat?*

When voluntary ingredient listing failed miserably, Professor Page and Anthony L. Young, a bright young lawyer and prime mover in the seminar, petitioned that cosmetic ingredient labeling be made mandatory under the Fair Packaging and Labeling Act. The law had been on the books for six years without being applied to cosmetics, even though the then FDA Commissioner, George P. Larrick, had testified in favor of cosmetic ingredient labeling under the bill at its Senate hearings, citing the need for consumer information.

Only when ingredient labeling became mandatory for all cosmetics did even the CTFA members comply. Although CTFA has planned a drive to urge more voluntary action from its members and the rest of the industry, there is little to indicate that the drive for company registration, formula disclosure, and adverse reaction or "product experience" reporting will be heeded by all segments of the industry until and unless it is made mandatory for the entire industry.

If the CTFA and the industry establishment wanted to expend their efforts more fruitfully, they might take Don Davis' suggestion that they reverse their lobbying efforts into requesting legislation that will make the voluntary program, even with its built-in industry-protective measures, mandatory. The Washington hierarchy might have to be treated for collective shock, *but it would be a heck of a public relations move for the cosmetic industry!*

QUESTIONS AND ANSWERS

A number of cosmetic company representatives have told me that their company's products have been approved by the FDA. Are cosmetics approved by the FDA?

I also have heard sales clerks and representatives, as well as one vice-president on television and another on radio, say that their products have been approved by the FDA. Do not be deceived by these statements, no matter who makes them. The FDA definitely does not approve cosmetic products. Nor does it test cosmetics before they are marketed as some would have you believe.

The only time the FDA tests cosmetic products is when they have been marketed and found or suspected to be contaminated, harmful, or otherwise deleterious.

What about some of the creams and lotions that are supposed to be all natural with no chemicals?

With literally unpreserved natural cosmetics, the hazard is the very real problem of contamination plus the more likely deterioration of the natural products—particularly when they must be transported and shelved for uncertain periods of time before the products are actually used.

One producer of "natural" cosmetics claimed its products could sustain a two-year shelf life while promoting the theory that "if they are good enough to eat, they should be good for your face." Conversely, I don't know how many consumers would risk eating or drinking a two-year-old egg, glass of milk, cucumber, avocado, grapefruit, papaya, strawberry, peach, orange, or any other perishable food that has been sitting on a shelf.

How many would enjoy *eating* lanolin, sperm whale oil, carnauba wax (advertised as being highly effective for waxing floors and cars), or even honeybees' wax— all of which are reportedly used in the "natural," "good-enough-to-eat" cosmetics?

If you want to go the "natural" route, I suggest you shop in your refrigerator and duplicate the egg shampoo, lemon rinse, olive-oil conditioner, avocado or grapefruit refresher, egg or honey mask, etc. You'll save money and avoid taking home embalmed produce or natural resting places for unfriendly bacteria.

‾ 24 ‾
Washington, D. C.

Of all FDA activities, the only FDA activity that
enjoys a lower priority than cosmetics within the
FDA is the Board of Tea Tasters, under the Tea
Importation Act.
—**Professor Joseph A. Page,**
Georgetown University Law Center

You begin by being angry at the so-called Division of
Cosmetics Technology, hidden away in a tiny corner of the Bureau of Foods, and wind up sympathizing with the plight of the
ragged buffeted orphan, all but rejected by the spread-eagled
enormity of the Food and Drug Administration and all but
unrecognized, unknown, and dismissed by the Big-Mama Department of Health and Human Services which is supposed to
take care of all its urchins.

The division's gravest failing—if a *sliver* can be called a
division—is its timid hesitation to ask for more than the miserly *7/10 of one percent* of the FDA budget that was doled to it
in the 1983 fiscal year ... to ask for sufficient funds and resources to do the job it is supposed to do.

In the face of the raging inflation of the past few years,

the $2.47 million allocated to the cosmetics program in 1983 is *$500,000 less* than the budget allocated to it in 1978. Ironically, while cosmetics are cavalierly dismissed in Washington, Nancy Reagan accompanied the president to Japan with her hairdresser as part of the entourage, reportedly paid for by the taxpayers.

There was also a new item on the 1983 budget chart—"Termination Costs"—which was allotted $3.451 million, or one million dollars more than the cosmetics division, which was expected to monitor and regulate a $12.5 *billion* industry. In other words, the cosmetics people in the FDA have been given a slingshot to use against a mammoth, increasingly impenetrable machine.

Consider the weight of dollars accessible to the cosmetic industry to overrun any threat of change or any attempt to hamper its uniquely privileged freewheeling style. Although the CTFA did not publish its budget in its 1983 annual report, the budget of just this one association would easily swallow that of FDA's cosmetic allotment.

As cosmetic-industry watcher Don Davis said, "If the CTFA needs another million dollars, all it has to do is to go to one or another of the major companies and they've got it."

How can the cosmetic industry come up with the funds so easily? Consider the profits. Most cosmetic ingredients cost pennies and can be translated into whatever the traffic will bear.

In a show of bravura, one major company offered to give me a price breakdown of a cream to justify its selling for $20. I, in turn, offered to include the breakdown in my report, only to be told, a few days later, that departmental consultation had resulted in a retraction of the company's offer. For some reason, the cream's price was then reduced to $15.

Contrast, too, the paltry national budget for overseeing an industry where $2.5 million a year can be considered to be just taxi fare. Take, for instance, the company that was praised for spending $20 million to introduce a product based on apricot kernels. Considering that FDA gave its cosmetic program only $1.855 million to operate for the entire year in 1980, the $20 million blowout on apricot kernels could have kept the division going almost a full decade.

Revlon surpassed the apricot kernelers with its reported $25 million advertising and promotion budget to be spent during one year of acquainting the public with its HDR shampoo and conditioner.

A look at some of the past promotional expenditures of cosmetics is similar to reading obituary notices. Many, if not most, of the cosmetics introduced with expensive fanfare have been speedily gone and forgotten. But as long as the companies can go back and mix up a batch of cream for a quarter a jar or a shampoo for fifteen cents a bottle and invest it with the mystique of an exotic herb or a "scientific breakthrough," all they need do is to sell the "new discoveries" at $25 or even $5 to continue to do well.

Meanwhile, back in Washington, D.C., the Division of Cosmetics Technology limps along trying to keep an industry in line when more than half the companies are not even known to it despite the grand-sounding voluntary registration program promoted by the CTFA.

When the CTFA told Senator Eagleton it had no objection to making its voluntary program mandatory, what was the FDA's commissioner's response? He protested that the division could not take on the "burden" because it didn't have the resources *instead of asking for the resources to do the job the FDA was mandated to do.*

So the charade goes on. The industry poaches on the FDA for people who can change sides and fight the FDA with its own weapons. When it can, the FDA reciprocates by hiring people from the industry, most of whom stay just long enough to learn whatever there is to learn so that they can return to the industry with an insider's knowledge to battle their former colleagues even more effectively. How else can those of the cosmetic industry manage to tie up dollars, time, and the meager manpower for almost two decades over a simple warning label on bubble bath?

The administration's transgression is the frequent politicized changing of the guard at the commissioner level and that of the Secretary of the Big-Mama Department of Health and Human Services. Then, of course, there was that 1981 Executive Order that compounded the Congress-passed Regulatory Flexibility Act, which, in effect, put industry in the driver's seat, thumbing its nose at regulations, would-be regulators, and, consequently, the taxpaying, industry-supporting public.

Since the cosmetics program of the FDA has been reduced to beggardom, it can do little more than accept handouts from the industry even though the burden of proof in any accusation of wrongdoing remains solidly with the FDA.

To avoid courting the long-delayed legislation needed to make the cosmetic program an effective division of the Food and Drug Administration, CTFA has compiled impressively presented technical guidelines, which it sells to its members and to nonmembers. According to Ed Kavanaugh, the comprehensive guidelines have become an industry bestseller.

Although, to my knowledge, the guidelines FDA provides for its inspectors are not sold, they are widely distributed and probably are even more widely read by cosmetic companies who may, one day, have a visit from an FDA inspector. Even so, over a three-year period of cosmetic company inspections, the FDA found that almost 90 percent of the 362 establishments inspected were deficient in at least one aspect of manufacture or control of cosmetics.

As Commissioner Arthur Hull Hayes, Jr., told the

CTFA 1983 conventioneers in Boca Raton, "While most of the deficiencies were what we may call 'typical,' they may nevertheless have influenced product integrity and possibly also product safety. More important yet, they could have been avoided without significant economic impact."

Insiders who knew the signals could recognize in the last phrase the directives from the administration that made the FDA tiptoe through its regulations.

Back in 1978, three years after the Senate-passed Cosmetic Safety Amendment died aborning, the U.S. General Accounting Office (GAO) delivered a blistering report by the Comptroller General to Congress. The 136-page report was headlined: "Lack of Authority Hampers Attempts To Increase Cosmetic Safety."

Among other things, the report cited the need for the FDA's issuance of Good Manufacturing Practices (GMP) for cosmetics. Said the GAO:

> Although FDA has established specific criteria, known as GMPs, for determining whether adequate methods, facilities, and controls are used in all phases of food and drug manufacture and distribution, it has not established such criteria for cosmetics. FDA uses such criteria in inspections of equipment, finished and unfinished materials, containers, manufacturing records, and laboratory controls.
>
> Under the FD&C Act, a cosmetic is deemed to be adulterated if it has been prepared, packed, or held under insanitary conditions whereby it may have become contaminated with filth or rendered injurious to health. Court decisions have established that it is unnecessary for the Government to prove that any product was actually contaminated. The courts have interpreted the term "insanitary conditions" to refer to conditions of manufacture or storage that would result, with reasonable possibility, in product contamination.
>
> GMP regulations would identify such conditions. Failure to manufacture or store cosmetics in accordance with GMP regulations would cause them to be deemed adulterated.

According to the Director of the Bureau of Foods' Office of Technology, although FDA has not established GMP regulations specifically applicable to cosmetics, it generally uses the food or drug GMP regulations as guidelines during inspections of cosmetic manufacturers. The drug GMP regulations state that manufacturers shall establish specifications for raw materials, test equipment for microbial contamination, establish specifications for finished products, test the effectiveness of preservative systems used in their products, and maintain batch records and an inventory control system adequate to facilitate a recall. According to a summary in its March 1975 Compliance Program Guidance Manual, FDA inspectors found during inspections that:

—Less than 33 percent of the establishments had raw material specifications.

—Less than 50 percent kept adequate batch records.

—Less than 15 percent tested equipment for microbial contamination.

—Only 30 percent had established finished product specifications (chemical, microbial, physical, etc.)

—Only 20 percent tested the effectiveness of preservative systems.

—Only 25 percent maintained inventory control systems adequate to facilitate a recall.

An attorney from FDA's Office of General Counsel told us that the food and drug GMP regulations cannot be applied to cosmetic inspections for enforcement purposes as regulations binding on cosmetics with the force of law. Although FDA has drafted GMP regulations for cosmetics, they had not been published in the Federal Register for comments as of March 1, 1978. Because FDA has not established GMP regulations for cosmetics, it has enforced the adulteration provisions of the act only when contamination could be proved.

In other words, the GAO was telling the FDA that, since it was not working smart, it was making its work harder.

For the next two years, various FDAers dutifully told various industry meetings that they were about to publish the GMPs for cosmetics. Then, suddenly, they were saying they saw no need to publish GMPs for the cosmetic industry.

In 1981, Heinz J. Eiermann, director of the Division of Cosmetics Technology, told the annual meeting of Independent Cosmetic Manufacturers and Distributors, a splinter trade association, there were several reasons for "a possible change in direction and publication of guidelines." The primary reasons were the change of climate in administrative Washington.

In 1983, Commissioner Hayes told CTFA conventioneers, in effect, to forget about FDA publishing the GMPs as the General Accounting Office had said they must. He suggested they use the FDA inspectors' poop sheet, instead, as their guide.

How successful was the new approach? According to the FDA, from 1976 to 1978, about 75 percent of a sample of over 300 firms inspected had deficiencies in their manufacturing practices. From July 1976 to September 1979, the percentage of deficiencies rose to 90 percent of the 362 cosmetic companies inspected. Between 46 and 62 percent, the highest deficiency rates, were found in raw material and product control practices. From 12 to 28 percent of the deficiencies were found in the areas of raw material storage and handling, general housekeeping, plant layout, and plant sanitation.

Even when violations or gross deficiencies were found during an inspection, the FDA has been notably lax in following up or assessing penalties.

The GAO reported that the FDA had failed to use its enforcement authority effectively in cases of serious or repeated violation. Its failure to do so "could indicate to the cosmetics industry that major violations of the law will be treated with minimum consequence."

In addition, the FDA failed to conduct timely follow-up inspections to assure that corrective action had been taken. Examples of the FDA laxity cited by the GAO included:

Firm A manufactures hair care and bath products and has estimated annual sales of between $500,000 and $1 million. FDA made three compliance inspections of this firm's manufacturing practices between August 1970 and March 1973. In each case the inspector found what he believed were major deficiencies in the firm's manufacturing practices. FDA had not inspected the firm's manufacturing practices since March 1973.

A summary of the August 1970 inspection stated that the firm was:

"* * * operating under conditions which may cause bacterial contamination of the finished product (Egg Shampoo). Poor housekeeping conditions such as pools of stagnant water, dirt, and debris on the floor in the manufacturing area and paint peeling from the ceiling directly over the mixing tank were found during the inspection. In addition, open unscreened door off the street to the manufacturing area could cause bacterial contamination of the finished product."

Inspection observations were discussed with the president of the firm, but no enforcement action was taken by the FDA. Although the president promised to correct the deficiencies, FDA did not make another inspection of the firm's manufacturing practices until January 1973.

During the January 1973 inspection, the firm was again found to be operating under poor sanitary conditions. A 41-point list was given to management pointing out conditions which could lead to bacterial or filth contamination of the firm's products, especially baby shampoo. The list of conditions included:

—Rodent excreta at several locations in the plant.

—A dead mouse in a storage closet, a live mouse in the firm's office.

—A "filthy, inadequate toilet facility" adjacent to the men's lunchroom with no wash basin and inoperable plumbing.

—Waste on the floor not confined to drain area.

—Foreign material in the "window" of the pipe feeding baby shampoo to the filler.

A post-inspection letter was sent to the manufacturer and re-inspection was scheduled for March 1973. Management replied to the letter and promised that corrections would be made.

However, the follow-up inspection revealed that the firm was still operating under unsanitary conditions. Many of the 59 deficiencies observed during this inspection were problems that had also been noted during the prior inspection. These conditions included:

—A dead, decomposed mouse on the storage room floor (according to the inspection report, "the same mouse noted in the January 1973 inspection").

—Rodent harborage areas throughout the plant.

—Sewers throughout the manufacturing areas left uncovered when not in use.

—A large accumulation of wash water and product waste on the floor.

—Equipment leaks allowing the product to seep out on the floor.

—An accumulation of a jelly-like substance in a crack in the floor near the product storage area.

All three inspections identified major deficiencies which the FDA inspector believed warranted regulatory action. Corrective action was again promised by the management after a discussion with FDA of the deficiencies. As of April 1978, no FDA follow-up had been made and no regulatory action taken.

Firm C is a nationally known cosmetic manufacturer having annual sales of between $5 million and $10 million. FDA inspected this firm's manufacturing practices twice between ... 1969 and 1975. Both inspections revealed major deficiencies, including poor manufacturing practices, use of hazardous ingredients, and microbial contamination in finished products. In addition, FDA examined 27 samples of the firm's products during the 7-year period. Only seven were found to be in compliance with the FD&C Act and FPLA [Fair Packaging and Labeling Act]. Of the 20 samples the laboratories found were not in compliance, 13 had major deficiences warranting regulatory action. Minor violations not requiring regulatory action were noted in the remaining samples.

In a June 1970 inspection, FDA noted several objectionable conditions, including deficiencies in manufacturing practices. Among the deficiencies were opened windows in the compounding area and lack of a sanitizing solution along the production lines. The need to correct the deficiencies was especially important in this case because samples collected at the time of the inspection revealed the presence of pathogenic *Pseudomonas* bacteria. The conditions noted could have contributed to the bacterial contamination of the firm's products.

In October 1973 the firm voluntarily recalled a shampoo containing bacterial contamination. FDA conducted a limited inspection to obtain information pertaining to the recall but did not inspect the firm's manufacturing practices.

However, during an October 1973 tour of the firm's plant, the Director and Deputy Director of the Division of Cosmetics Technology noticed what they considered deficiencies in the firm's manufacturing practices. They noted that:

"Microbiological control facilities were essentially nonexistent and demonstrated poor housekeeping. Control specifications were minimal at best. Based on remarks made by * * * [company officials] guidelines for proper preservation of products were inadequate, and microbiological testing appeared to be minimal."

During a November 1975 inspection, many objectionable conditions were again noted in the manufacturing area. The inspection disclosed that not all raw materials were identified, some raw materials were stored under conditions whereby they may become contaminated, and manufacturing equipment was uncovered in an area having open unscreened windows. A list of 18 deficiencies was discussed with the manufacturer. Management promised corrections for most of the deficiencies, but in other cases when the deficiencies would result in the product being exposed to unsanitary conditions, management felt that the deficiences were not significant and did not agree to take corrective action.

No deficiencies were noted in manufacturing practices during a follow-up inspection in October 1976. However, when the inspector asked to review the firm's microbiological test data, the firm denied FDA access to the data until the request was considered by the firm's lawyers. Consent was never received and FDA made no further attempts to obtain the test data. As of March 1978 no further action had been taken by the FDA.

According to the GAO, the FDA's efforts were further limited "because FDA lacks adequate legislative authority to (1) obtain access to a manufacturer's production and other records and (2) assess civil penalties for violations of the cosmetic provisions of the FD&C Act."

The lack of legislative authority to obtain access to records is the biggest stumbling block to any meaningful regulation. When I asked an FDA representative how safety or anything else could be substantiated without access to records, there was a long silence.

Then I was told, "Well, we can request records, but they don't have to give them to us. Then, the burden of proof is on us to prove that the safety of the product was not substantiated."

Is it any mystery why *not one action* has surfaced against any of the hundreds of thousands of cosmetic products on the market that are riding under the presumption of safety substantiation?

The idea that the "threat" of *safety substantiation* is keeping the entire cosmetic industry as honest and true as the truest boy scout is a monumental practical joke on an uninformed public.

Behind the smokescreen of "safety substantiation," the

industry has dealt the consumers the joker in the pack . . . and the industry is holding all the aces.

Sitting in on the many industry meetings, briefings, seminars, and symposia, it is understandable why the reappearing industry lawyers repeatedly counsel industry members that no FDA inspector or representative has a legal right to see any production record or records of any kind. All an inspector can do is "eyeball" the premises and take samples of the products.

If a claim for safety substantiation is challenged by the FDA, it is the FDA that must substantiate and prove its challenge, and not the company questioned. Apparently, all the company has to do is to assure the FDA that is has the substantiating records in its file cabinet and never open the file cabinet drawer.

Of course, the FDA can always chase the products after they've been marketed in interstate commerce, and it could cite deficiencies on inspections, which have become abbreviated in an effort to inspect more than the token number of known cosmetic firms. Even so, the GAO pointed out that the FDA had taken regulatory action in only about 20 percent of the violations the FDA determined warranted such action. Of the violations found in the agency's meager haphazard sweep, 80 percent escaped without *any* action being taken.

The GAO concluded: "Because of the low priority of the cosmetics program, it is essential that FDA effectively use the limited resources available for market surveillance and enforcement. By establishing GMPs for cosmetics, FDA could provide guidance to FDA inspectors and manufacturers in identifying conditions which might result in a product becoming contaminated and form a firm basis for enforcement action. However, establishment of GMPs will not have a significant effect unless FDA insures that prompt and effective enforcement action is taken when violations are identified."

As for Congress, the GAO addressed it on the front cover of its report:

> The Congress should authorize the Food and Drug Administration to require cosmetic manufacturers to prove the safety of their products. Because the agency does not have enough authority to effectively regulate cosmetics, products are being marketed which may pose a hazard to consumers. About 125 ingredients available for use in cosmetics are suspected of causing cancer, and about 25 are suspected of causing birth defects. Although many of the reported adverse effects have not been verified, 30 of the ingredients are known to cause cancer in humans or animals or contain impurities known to cause cancer. The ability of these ingredients to cause toxic effects through cosmetic use has not been determined.

> Manufacturers do not have to determine the safety of their products before selling them or tell the Food and Drug Administration what ingredients are used in them. Many manufacturers have not voluntarily given such information to the agency. As a result, a hazardous cosmetic can be marketed until the Food and Drug Administration obtains information to prove that the product may be injurious to users.

In the 1970s, the word around Capitol Hill and environs was that there had to be "thalidomide" in cosmetics before Congress would act to pass any legislation that would make cosmetics—the sales of which, Senator Eagleton said, totaled more than prescription drugs and over-the-counter drugs combined, and of which the units sold, according to CTFA, were surpassed only by food—a legitimate partner to food and drugs in the so-called Food, Drug, and Cosmetic Act.

Well, there have been thalidomides in cosmetics. How else would one classify forty babies dead after being dusted with talcum powder containing unnecessary and unwarranted hexachlorophene that was promoted throughout the nation as a cosmetic ingredient "good" for the entire family? Did the press fail in not featuring photographs of forty lifeless infants on their front pages as it did with the photographs of the tragically deformed "thalidomide" infants? Must we be shocked by children burned to mutilation from hazardously inflammable colognes packaged in miniature model automobiles, promoted for the Christmas holidays and destined to be mistaken for toys? Are there enough investigative reporters to uncover the tragedies paid off in out-of-court settlements in which all participants are sworn to silence? And which publication, eager for more and more cosmetic advertising, would dare publish these reports?

In the 1980s, when more and more cosmetics are being exposed as being dangerously contaminated with potentially blinding pseudomonas, with cancer-causing nitrosamines, and with mutagenic ingredients, the word heard on Capitol Hill is that there have to be "bodies in the streets" before Congress is moved to take another look and have another hearing on the need for cosmetic safety and to legitimize the phrase that strikes fear in the profit-heavy cosmetic industry and *real* hope in the taxpaying consumers—*premarket testing.*

Must the American consumers who have come to expect dry armpits and talcumed babies continue to be paying guinea pigs simply because they would like to look and smell a little better?

Now that cosmetics, and what men prefer to call "toiletries," have become part of our everyday life, should they not be treated as the staples they have become, with the premarket checks and consumer safeguards appropriate to staples used by the entire population every day of our lives?

In these "enlightened" 1980s, on the threshold of the twenty-first century, it remains to convince the still unconvinced—or, more likely, *the unaware*—in Washington.

References

Ames, Bruce N.; Kammen, H. O.; Yamasaki. "Hair Dyes Are Mutagenic: Identification of a Variety of Mutagenic Ingredients." *Proceedings of the National Academy of Sciences of the United States of America.* June 1975.

CIR & Industry: A Sourcebook. Washington, D.C. The Cosmetic, Toiletry and Fragrance Association, Inc. 1982.

Congressional Record. Washington, D.C.

Cosmetic Injury Reports from Consumers as Reported to Division of Cosmetics Technology. Washington, D.C.: Food and Drug Administration.

Cosmetic Insiders' Report. New York, N.Y.: HBJ Newsletter Bureau.

Cosmetic Recalls and Seizures by the Food and Drug Administration. Washington, D.C.: Food and Drug Administration.

Cosmetics, Science and Technology, edited by Edward Sagarin. New York: Interscience Publishers, Inc., 1957.

CTFA Cosmetic Ingredient Dictionary. Washington, D.C.: The Cosmetic, Toiletry and Fragrance Association, Inc., 1982.

CTFA Cosmetic Journal. Washington, D.C.: The Cosmetic, Toiletry and Fragrance Association.

CTFA International Resource Manual. Washington, D.C.: The Cosmetic, Toiletry and Fragrance Association, Inc., 1982.

CTFA Technical Guidelines. Washington, D.C.: The Cosmetic, Toiletry and Fragrance Association, Inc., 1981.

Drug and Cosmetic Industry. Cleveland, Ohio: Harcourt Brace Jovanovich Publications.

Drug Industry Act of 1962, Hearings before the Committee on Interstate and Foreign Commerce. House of Representatives, 87th Congress, Second Session.

Executive Newsletter. Washington, D.C.: The Cosmetic, Toiletry and Fragrance Association, Inc.

FDA Consumer. Rockville, Maryland: Food and Drug Administration.

FDA Quarterly Activities Report. Washington, D.C.: U.S. Department of Health and Human Services, Public Health Service, Food and Drug Administration.

FDA Talk Paper. Rockville, Maryland: Food and Drug Administration.

FDC Reports—"The Pink Sheet." Chevy Chase, Maryland: F-D-C Reports, Inc.

FDC Reports—"The Rose Sheet." Chevy Chase, Maryland: F-D-C Reports, Inc.

Federal Hazardous Substances Labeling Act, Hearing before a Subcommittee of the Committee on Interstate and Foreign Commerce. House of Representatives, 86th Congress, Second Session.

Federal Register. Washington, D.C.

Federal Trade Commission Decisions, Findings, Orders and Stipulations. Washington, D.C.: Federal Trade Commission.

Food and Drug Administration Annual Report. Washington, D.C.: Department of Health and Human Services, Public Health Service, Food and Drug Administration.

Food and Drug Administration Weekly Report of Seizures, Prosecutions, Injunctions, Field Corrections, and Recalls. Washington, D.C.: Food and Drug Administration.

FTC News. Washington, D.C.: Federal Trade Commission.

Hearings before the House Select Committee to Investigate the Use of Chemicals in Foods and Cosmetics. House of Representatives, 82nd Congress, Second Session, 1952.

Hearings before the Subcommittee on Oversight and Investigations of the Committee on Interstate and Foreign Commerce. Cancer-Causing Chemicals—Part 1, Safety of Cosmetics and Hair Dyes, 95th Congress, Second Session, January 23 and 26; February 2 and 3, 1978.

HHS News. Washington, D.C.: U.S. Department of Health and Human Services.

Import Alert, Regulatory Procedure Manual. Washington, D.C.: Field Compliance Branch, Food and Drug Administration.

International Cosmetic Regulations. Brussels, Belgium: Sponsored by the International Federation of Societies of Cosmetic Chemists Conference, 1977.

The Johns Hopkins Center for Alternatives to Animal Testing. Baltimore, Maryland: Office of Public Affairs, The Johns Hopkins Medical Institutions.

Journal of the American Medical Association. Chicago, Illinois: The American Medical Association.

Long, James M. *CTFA Labeling Manual.* Washington, D.C.: The Cosmetic, Toiletry and Fragrance Association, Inc.

The Merck Index. New York: Merck & Co., 1960.

Notices of Judgement under the Federal Food, Drug, and Cosmetic Act. Washington, D.C.: Food and Drug Administration.

Packard, Vance, *The Hidden Persuaders.* New York: David McKay Co., Inc. 1957.

Physicians' Desk Reference. Oradell, N.J.: Medical Economics Company.

Report to the Congress by the Comptroller General of the United States. Washington, D.C.: United States Accounting Office, August 8, 1978.

Requirements of Laws and Regulations Enforced by the U.S. Food and Drug Administration. Rockville, Maryland: U.S. Department of Health, Education, and Welfare, Public Health Service, Food and Drug Administration, 1980.

Soap/Cosmetics/Chemical Specialties. New York: MacNair-Dorland Company, Inc.

Spencer, Peter S.; Sterman, Arnold B.; Bischoff, Monica; Horoupian, Dikran; Foster, Grover V. *Abstract: Transactions American Neurological Association, Experimental Myelin Disease and Ceroid Accumulation Produced by the Fragrance Compound Acetyl Ethyl Tetramethyl Tetralin (A.E.T.T.).*

Stabile, Toni. *Cosmetics: Trick or Treat?.* New York: Hawthorn Books, Inc., 1966; Arco Publishing Company, Inc., 1967; Arc Books, 1969.

Stabile, Toni. *Cosmetics: The Great American Skin Game.* New York: Ballantine Books, 1973; Charter Books, 1979.

Stabile, A. D. "The Outrageous Cost of Facial 'Beauty'." *Reader's Digest,* Novemeber 1960.

Stark, Dennis M. "Progress in Alternatives to Animal Testing," presented at Seminar for Science Writers, The Rockefeller University, New York, N.Y., June 2, 1983.

Swartz, Harry. *How to Master Your Allergy.* New York: Thomas Nelson & Sons, 1961.

Today's Health. Chicago, Illinois: The American Medical Association.

Index